GUIDE TO THE GUIDELINES

Volume 2

GI Infection, Inflammation, and Bleeding

Brennan Spiegel, MD, MSHS, FACG

and

Hetal A. Karsan, MD, FACG

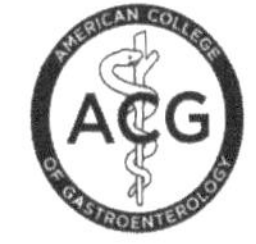

This book is intended as an educational resource for healthcare professionals and should not replace individual clinical judgment. The authors and the American College of Gastroenterology (ACG) make no guarantees regarding the accuracy or completeness of the information presented and assume no liability for any errors, omissions, or consequences arising from the application of the content. Clinicians are encouraged to consult relevant guidelines directly and use their discretion in applying information from this book to patient care.

Published by The American College of Gastroenterology
11333 Woodglen Drive, Suite 100
North Bethesda, MD 20852
www.gi.org
Email: info@gi.org

Contents

Preface: Know Your Guidelines! 5

Chapter One: The Inflamed Pathways 9

Chapter Two: The Unwelcome Guests 89

Chapter Three: When the River Runs Red 165

Acknowledgments 243

About the Authors 244

References..247

Abbreviations..259

KNOW YOUR GUIDELINES!

"What do the ACG guidelines say?"

If you're a practicing gastroenterologist or hepatologist, then that's an excellent question. It's a question you probably ask yourself every day you are in clinic. It's a question that determines how best to diagnose, treat, and deliver the highest quality care for patients with digestive diseases. Bottom line is this: you really must know the guidelines!

Of course, the best way to know the guidelines is to read them. As of this writing, the American College of Gastroenterology (ACG) has published over 75 guidelines covering diseases of the esophagus, to disorders the anorectum, to, well, just about everywhere else between the poles of the alimentary canal. These documents are pure gold. They lay out, in evidence-based splendor, the key recommendations that govern clinical practice in our field. They are required reading.

But let's be fair about something. Reading through 75+ guidelines encompassing well over 4,000 pages of text and drawing from over 10,000 citations is not easy sledding. By the time you reach the end of the guidelines you probably need to start over because (a) you forgot some things, (b) the guidelines are periodically revised, and (c) new guidelines are constantly in the works.

That's why we wrote this book. As a former Editor-in-Chief of *The American Journal of Gastroenterology* (B.S.) and former Editor of the Journal's "Red Section" (H.K.), we have observed a strong desire among clinicians to learn the guidelines in efficient, accessible, and fun ways. We discovered that our most popular Journal podcasts were those about the ACG guidelines and the most successful Red Section columns were authored by senior clinicians who interpreted the guidelines through an expert lens shaped by years of practice.

We got to thinking: wouldn't it be handy to have a "guide to the guidelines" that digested (pun intended) the 4,000 pages of ACG documents into a concise, entertaining, and useful review of the most salient pearls and insights? We imagined a resource that would reflect the accessible style of our AJG podcasts with the pragmatic lessons in the most popular Red Section columns. Also, because clinicians learn by example, we figured that a vignette-based journey through the guidelines would bring the ACG material to life in ways that a typical textbook might fall short (peeps love to learn from vignettes). That led to the book you are reading now.

Here's how we structured Guide to the Guidelines, which we call G2G for short: We mapped each of the ACG guidelines into 3 major topics. Each topic composes 1 of 3 volumes for the G2G series. You are now holding Volume II, titled *GI Infections, Inflammation, and Bleeding*. In Chapter 1, "The Inflamed Pathways," we summarize all the guidelines on Crohn's disease, ulcerative colitis, and celiac disease. Chapter 2, "The Unwelcome Guests," reviews the guidelines on various GI infections, including *Helicobacter pylori, Clostridioides difficile*, and acute infectious diarrheal illnesses. Finally, in Chapter 3, "When the River Runs Red," we cover the guidelines on upper GI and ulcer bleeding, lower GI bleeding, management of anticoagulants and antiplatelet drugs during acute GI bleeding, and colon ischemia.

If you haven't already seen Volume I, titled *Bread and Butter GI*, go check it out! There, we cover common luminal topics that comprise everyday practice for the general gastroenterologist, including the neurogastroenterology and motility guidelines on irritable bowel syndrome (IBS), small intestinal bacterial overgrowth, dyspepsia, constipation, gastroparesis, and benign anorectal disorders. Volume I also reviews the key esophagus guidelines including gastroesophageal reflux disease, Barrett's esophagus, esophageal eosinophilia, and achalasia. Finally, in the inaugural G2G volume we covered prevention and treatment of luminal tumors, including colorectal cancer screening and surveillance guidelines, GI polyposis syndromes, hereditary GI cancer syndromes, gastric premalignant conditions, and submucosal masses. Give it a read if you haven't already ;-)

In Volume III, we will leave the main luminal highway and head towards the extraluminal onramps, including the pancreas and biliary system. There, we'll review the ACG guidelines on biliary strictures, use of endoscopic retrograde cholangiopancreatography (ERCP) and endoscopic ultrasound (EUS), pancreatic cysts, pancreatitis, and primary sclerosing cholangitis. Finally, we end with that big organ up top: the liver. We'll review the guidelines on alcoholic liver diseases, focal liver lesions, hemochromatosis, acute liver failure, hepatic and mesenteric circulation, abnormal liver tests, drug induced liver injury, pregnancy and liver disease, and nutrition in liver disease. Yep, that's a lot of guidelines!

Each G2G chapter includes carefully selected vignettes designed to illustrate key concepts from the guidelines, followed by a conversation-style discussion written to keep you awake and alert. As you read these discussions, you'll notice that we highlight specific points along the margin that we think are especially noteworthy. Then, following each chapter, we provide multiple-choice questions to test your knowledge of the material. We prepared questions that highlight information we believe is most vital to ensure high quality care, as judged by our nearly 50 years of combined experience managing GI and liver patients in both academic and private practice settings (yikes, we're getting old). We also worked with the authors of each ACG guideline to ensure our treatment of their document is accurate and thank them all for their time and commitment ot this ACG project. We hope you find the discussions and questions to be both enjoyable and useful.

Because the ACG guidelines are constantly revised and updated, the book you are now reading will eventually become outdated. In fact, it might already be outdated! That's the nature of guidelines. It's important to keep up with the latest recommendations because they often change meaningfully as scientific evidence emerges. We will continue to update this book to ensure it remains modern and accurate. Life is a work in progress.

We hope you enjoy reading the G2G series as much as we enjoyed writing it. If nothing else, preparing this resource in partnership with the ACG helped us learn the guidelines and we trust it will help you, too.

Brennan Spiegel, MD, MSHS, FACG
Professor of Medicine and Public Health
Gourrich Chair in Digital Health Ethics
Director of Health Services Research,
Cedars-Sinai
Director, Cedars-Sinai Master's Degree
Program in Health Delivery Science

Hetal A. Karsan, MD, FACG
Chair of Credentials Committee, ACG
International Governor, ACG
Chair of Medical Education,
United Digestive
Adjunct Professor of Medicine, Emory
University

CHAPTER ONE

THE INFLAMED PATHWAYS

Understanding Colitis: Spanning IBD to Celiac

If you're like us, keeping up with the latest in managing inflammatory bowel diseases (IBD) feels overwhelming. With new biologics, clinical trials, and anti-inflammatory mechanisms constantly emerging, it's challenging to stay updated. Unless you're an "IBD-ologist" (a term we all use, even if it's not in the Oxford English Dictionary), it can be tough to keep track of the latest on Crohn's disease and ulcerative colitis (UC). Thankfully, the ACG IBD guidelines have us covered. In this chapter, we've distilled the critical points from those comprehensive documents.

We can't cover everything about IBD—that would take several volumes—but we will at least cover the basics. Already an IBD-ologist? Great! Feel free to skip to Chapter 2, or go back to Volume I and read all about IBS—we know you can brush up on IBS too.

IBD goes beyond Crohn's and UC. Celiac disease is also an inflammatory bowel disease. So, we also cover the ACG celiac guidelines in this chapter. Microscopic colitis is another IBD, but the ACG has no guidelines on that topic yet. Hint to the Practice Parameters Committee: unmet need alert!

Enjoy Chapter 1, and when you're done, check out the quiz at the end of the chapter to see how much you've learned. Or take the quiz first and then go back to fill in the blanks—whatever floats your boat!

Case 1.1: Ileitis Insights

A 23-year-old woman with a body mass index of 34 kg/m^2 presents to your open access colonoscopy clinic with a 6-month history of right lower quadrant abdominal pain and sporadic joint discomfort. She reports no significant changes in diet or activity level, yet she has experienced recent unexplained weight loss and intermittent fevers. Despite maintaining a robust appetite, her pain now is disrupting sleep and daily activities, while fatigue has become common.

Chart review indicates the patient was found to have tenderness in the right lower quadrant but no guarding or rebound. Initial labs showed elevated inflammatory markers, including high erythrocyte sedimentation rate (ESR), C-reactive protein (CRP), and platelet count. A magnetic resonance enterography (MRE) suggested inflammation of the terminal ileum.

You now perform colonoscopy which reveals terminal ileitis and right-sided colitis. To complicate matters, a perianal fistula is identified on inspection of the anus (which, by the way, should probably have been found on an earlier rectal exam, but you go back to the chart and discover nobody ever documented a rectal exam because "colonoscopy was scheduled anyway"... but we digress).

Know your guidelines!

1. Is there enough evidence to make the diagnosis of Crohn's disease at this time? If not, what other tests are indicated?

2. Assuming this is Crohn's disease, what specific risk factors does this patient have that portend a high risk for progressive and severe disease?

Case 1.1: What do the guidelines say?

Source: ACG 2018 Crohn's Disease Guidelines[1]

Crohn's disease is a form of IBD that can affect any part of the gastrointestinal tract (mouth to anus), although it most commonly involves the terminal ileum and colon, as seen in this case. Its epidemiology has been of particular interest in recent decades due to increasing incidence and prevalence in both adult and pediatric populations worldwide.

The most recent data from the Centers for Disease Control (CDC) reveals that the U.S. prevalence of IBD is between 2.4 and 3.1 milllion people.[2] Among those with Crohn's, onset typically occurs between the ages of 15 and 30, with a second, smaller peak occurring in individuals between 50 and 80 years of age. So, this patient is right in the sweet spot for the first peak of Crohn's disease onset.

The risk factors for developing Crohn's disease are multifactorial, involving a combination of genetic predisposition, environmental factors, and alterations in the gut microbiome. There is a recognized familial pattern, with a higher risk observed in first-degree relatives of affected individuals.

For now, let's start by focusing on how to make the diagnosis. The issue here is that many conditions can mimic Crohn's disease, so it's vital to secure the diagnosis with sufficient probability before starting treatment. The last thing you want is to miss an infection and then launch headlong into IBD management with steroids, immune modulators, or biologics.

In this case, the patient has evidence of terminal ileitis. This definitely suggests Crohn's, but let's not forget about the long list of other conditions that can affect the terminal ileum. **Figure 1.1**, below, provides a mnemonic to help you remember some of the other causes.

Figure 1.1. *A memory aid to learn the causes of terminal ileitis. They spell out the words "CROHN'S MAP"*

C rohn's disease/ **C** hurg-Strauss syndrome
R adiation enteritis
O vergrowth of bacteria (e.g., Yersinia, TB)
H istoplasmosis / **H** enoch-Schönlein purpura
N SAID-induced enteropathy / **N** eoplasms (e.g., lymphoma)
S arcoid / **S** almonella typhi or enteriditis

M eckel's diverticulitis
A ctinomycosis / **A** utoimmune (e.g., Bechet's)
P arasites (e.g., cryptosporidiosis) / **P** soriasis

For instance, an infection with *Yersinia enterocolitica* can often be mistaken for Crohn's disease. *Yersinia* can cause an extended period of diarrhea, much longer than what's typical for common pathogens. Because this diarrhea can persist for weeks, it might trigger concerns about chronic conditions like IBD. Additionally, *Yersinia* can lead to symptoms such as erythema nodosum and reactive arthritis, both of which are also seen in IBD, adding to the diagnostic confusion. Moreover, *Yersinia* has a penchant for the terminal ileum and cecum, which are frequent targets of Crohn's. This overlap can complicate the diagnosis further, so it's vital to always look for enteric infections like *Yersinia* before settling on a diagnosis of Crohn's disease.

Yersina enterocolitica can mimic Crohn's

Given the similarities with other conditions, diagnosing Crohn's presents a real challenge. There's no one-size-fits-all test; instead, diagnosis mandates a careful consideration of various signs, symptoms, and test outcomes. The ACG guidelines suggest testing for fecal pathogens, *Clostridioides difficile*, and fecal calprotectin. Fecal calprotectin is particularly valuable for differentiating between IBS and IBD,[3] a topic we covered in *G2G Volume 1* (a good reason to revisit that discussion). Since the current vignette did not mention any of these tests, they should be checked before confirming the diagnosis of Crohn's disease. Of course, we also need biopsies and microscopy, looking for signs of architectural distortion, granulomata, Paneth cell metaplasia, and other evidence of chronic inflammation characteristic of Crohn's.

A complete blood count might reveal anemia or an elevated platelet count (as seen here), the latter indicating inflammation. Non-cardiac CRP levels can be telling, especially during active flares. Since CRP's half-life is brief, any elevation signals recent inflammation.[4] While CRP helps differentiate IBS from IBD, ESR doesn't offer the same clarity, though it's often high in IBD cases. It is important to note that up to 40% of IBD patients with mild inflammation may have normal CRP and ESR levels, limiting the diagnostic utility of these markers. Remember, diagnosing IBD, especially Crohn's, is a holistic puzzle. Don't rely on any one bit of evidence to rule-in, or rule-out, IBD. Let's go through some of the other tidbits we might use to cinch the diagnosis.

Genetic Testing. Although genetic testing is an area of great interest in Crohn's disease, the ACG guidelines indicate that testing isn't yet primetime for routine clinical use. Despite identifying over 200 genetic loci linked to IBD, with more than 70 of these specifically associated with Crohn's susceptibility, these insights still remain more academic than clinical. Large-scale genome-wide association studies have illuminated the roles of certain genes in Crohn's disease, such as NOD2, the IL-23 receptor, and ATG16L1 (go ahead and memorize that). These genes are integral to our innate immune response and the maintenance of the intestinal barrier.

While these genetic variants offer a glimpse into the pathophysiology of Crohn's, their diagnostic value in practice is limited. No single genetic variant is prevalent enough in those with Crohn's to serve as a reliable diagnostic marker. Moreover, the prevalence of these genetic markers can vary across different racial and ethnic groups. For instance, variants in NOD2 and IL23R are rare in East Asian populations.

Some genetic variants, like those in NOD2, are linked to more severe disease courses, including ileal involvement and an increased likelihood of requiring surgery. However, despite the availability of commercial testing for these variants, their application in clinical settings has been minimal. The field is moving towards a future where genetic testing might guide therapy choices more precisely, but for now, the ACG guidelines explain that genetic testing remains a research tool rather than a clinical necessity in diagnosing Crohn's disease. Thus, it's not indicated in this patient to make the diagnosis.

Serological Studies. The same thing applies to serological markers. In the quest to distinguish Crohn's disease from UC and normal controls, serological markers like ANCA (anti-neutrophil cytoplasmic antibodies) and ASCA (anti-saccharomyces cerevisiae antibodies) have garnered attention over the years. ANCA is more commonly associated with UC, while ASCA is more frequently positive in patients with Crohn's disease.[5] These markers offer a glimpse into the complex immunological landscape of IBD, potentially aiding in differentiating between forms of IBD when the clinical picture is murky. Indeed, the whole notion of IBD collapsing into "UC" and "CD" is pretty archaic; we now know there are many intermediary conditions along the spectrum between these archetypal diseases. However, despite the promise of serological studies in IBD, the ACG guidelines do not yet recommend these studies for routine use. Rather, these tests are considered supportive—not definitive—in diagnosing IBD. The guidelines emphasize that, while informative, ANCA and ASCA should not replace clinical judgment and comprehensive evaluation.

Endoscopy. Ileocolonoscopy with biopsies plays a crucial role in diagnosing Crohn's disease, aimed at documenting disease distribution and severity. Yet, while over 80% of IBD patients show mucosal involvement within colonoscopy's reach, traditional imaging like small bowel follow-through may misrepresent ileal disease. Hence, direct ileal examination is preferred for a comprehensive diagnosis.[6]

Upper endoscopy is recommended only for patients with upper GI symptoms, considering the low prevalence of Crohn's in the upper GI tract. Visible and histologic inflammation is common, even in asymptomatic patients, but often lacks clinical significance.

Video capsule endoscopy can often be a valuable diagnostic adjunct for small bowel Crohn's, especially where traditional imaging falls short.[7] It surpasses small bowel barium studies, CT enterography, and ileocolonoscopy in diagnostic yield for suspected Crohn's. However, its specificity remains under debate,[8] and a patency capsule or imaging must precede it to minimize capsule retention risk.

Deep enteroscopy, though not routinely used, can offer additional insights where biopsy or sampling of small bowel tissue is necessary for diagnosis. Techniques like single and double balloon enteroscopy have shown high diagnostic yields, but their invasive nature suggests they should be reserved for specific cases requiring tissue diagnosis or therapeutic intervention.

Imaging Studies. Small bowel imaging is a cornerstone in the initial diagnostic approach for suspected Crohn's disease, with both computed tomography enterography (CTE) and MRE (which stands for "Meal Ready to Eat" in the military, but that's another story...) offering high sensitivity in detecting small bowel involvement.[9] MRE, devoid of radiation risks, is favored for

MRE is generally preferred over CTE for younger patients and/or those in need of recurrent imaging

younger patients and those requiring frequent monitoring, and that's why it was used in this case. The choice between CTE and MRE largely depends on the institution's expertise and the patient's specific clinical picture.

Up to half of the patients with active small bowel Crohn's may have inflammation that eludes ileocolonoscopy,[10] highlighting the importance of imaging for identifying both inflammation and complications like strictures and fistulas. CTE's high sensitivity and MRE's comparable performance, along with their ability to visualize beyond the terminal ileum, make them invaluable. Both modalities can detect inflammation, aiding in treatment evaluation and prognostication. Given the cumulative radiation exposure associated with repeated CTE exams, MRE is preferred for ongoing surveillance, especially among younger patients and those with complex disease needing recurrent imaging.

For perianal Crohn's disease, magnetic resonance imaging (MRI) of the pelvis and endoscopic ultrasound excel in detailing perirectal complications, such as fistulas and abscesses, which is essential for surgical planning and therapeutic management. Their high diagnostic accuracy supports their use in both initial evaluation and monitoring the effectiveness of interventions. We'll come back to perirectal disease in a later vignette, so stay tuned.

In cases of suspected intra-abdominal abscesses, the guidelines emphasize that CTE and MRE again prove highly accurate, aiding in preoperative planning and potentially reducing post-surgical complications through guided drainage. More on that, too, later in the book.

Risk Factors for Disease Progression. Lastly, let's quickly review the risk factors for disease progression. This patient, regrettably, ticks several boxes for high-risk indicators. Factors signaling a heightened risk include a younger age at onset, concurrent involvement of both the ileum and colon, presence of perianal disease, and initial presentation with complications such as penetration or stricture formation. Additionally, those with increased visceral fat are, on average, more prone to experience aggressive disease courses.[11] Given this patient's profile, which aligns with several high-risk characteristics, vigilant monitoring and an appropriately aggressive treatment plan are imperative, topics we'll explore through various vignettes in this chapter. For a quick reference on these risk factors, see **Table 1.1** below.

Table 1.1. *Risk factors for progressive disease burden in Crohn's disease*

Young age at diagnosis
Initial extensive bowel involvement
Ileal/ileocolonic involvement
Perianal/severe rectal disease
Penetrating or stenosis disease phenotype
Visceral adiposity

Case 1.2: Assessing Crohn's Severity

A 32-year-old man is referred to you for management of Crohn's disease. He has experienced recurrent diarrhea, abdominal pain, and around 15% weight loss over the past 3 months. He reports that his quality of life has suffered as a result of his disease, although he has not required hospitalization or intravenous hydration.

Physical exam reveals tenderness in the right lower quadrant, without any palpable masses. No fistulae are noted on rectal exam. A complete blood count shows mild anemia and an elevated platelet count. CRP levels and fecal calprotectin are also elevated. MRE reveals thickening of the terminal ileum with enhanced mucosal contrast uptake, but no signs of stricturing or fistula formation.

Know your guidelines!

1. Based on the clinical findings and diagnostic workup described, how would you rate the level of disease activity?

2. What factors did you consider when evaluating disease activity?

3. How should disease activity be monitored over time?

Case 1.2: What do the guidelines say?

Source: ACG 2018 Crohn's Disease Guidelines[1]

In IBD, assessing clinical disease activity is crucial yet challenging, with no universally accepted "gold standard." Disease activity is categorized into four levels: remission, mild, moderate, and severe, based on a mix of clinical symptoms, the disease's impact on quality of life, and any complications arising from the disease or its treatment.[12] In this case, it's clear the patient is not in remission, so the question is how best to classify disease activity along the mild-to-severe spectrum.

"Mild" disease manifests in patients who maintain their normal daily activities and diet without significant complications like obstruction, fever, abdominal mass, or dehydration. Symptoms may include diarrhea and abdominal pain, often with a slight increase in serum CRP levels, and less than 10% weight loss. This level of disease activity typically has a minimal impact on quality of life and aligns with a Crohn's Disease Activity Index (CDAI) score of 150–220.[1] The components of the CDAI are listed in **Table 1.2**. In the current vignette, the patient has lost 15% body weight and has a decreased quality of life, suggesting disease activity beyond the "mild" level of severity.

On the flip side, "severe disease" is marked by cachexia, substantial weight loss, and complications such as obstruction or intra-abdominal abscesses. Patients with severe disease often require hospitalization, even after aggressive therapy, corresponding to a CDAI score of over 450.[1] The patient in the vignette does not have evidence of these findings, suggesting he falls somewhere below the severe level of disease.

Table 1.2. *Components of the CDAI.*[13] *The sum of these components is used to calculate a total score. This index, while widely used in clinical trials and research, is less commonly applied in routine clinical practice due to its complexity, but it's good to at least know the components of the CDAI.*

Number of liquid or very soft stools over the past 7 days
Abdominal pain rating over the past seven days, scored from 0 (no pain) to 3 (severe pain)
General well-being, self-assessed over the past 7 days, on a scale from 0 (well) to 4 (terrible)
Presence of complications related to Crohn's disease, such as fistulas, abscesses, fevers, etc., with each complication contributing a specific score
Use of loperamide or opiates for diarrhea
Presence of an abdominal mass (as determined by physical examination), with scoring based on size and tenderness
Hematocrit value, adjusted for gender, to account for anemia
Body weight, compared to ideal body weight, to assess weight loss

"Moderate" disease activity falls between these two extremes, where symptoms are more pronounced than in mild disease but without the severe complications or need for hospitalization characteristic of severe disease. It's important to note that the level of symptomatic disease activity doesn't always match the disease's natural progression. In the current case, the ability to maintain hydration, lack of recent hospitalizations, and lack of intraabdominal abscesses on imaging all argue against severe disease. On the other hand, the weight loss and impact on quality of life indicate this is beyond mild disease.

While the CDAI doesn't need to be formally calculated at every visit—typically, this level of assessment is reserved for clinical trials or detailed evaluations—the ACG guidelines do suggest categorizing patients within a spectrum from remission to severe disease activity.

It's important to reassess and clearly document this classification in the patient's chart during each visit.

The guidelines recommend various ways to monitor disease severity over time. Fecal markers like lactoferrin and calprotectin can be used as effective indicators. These markers are pretty good at reflecting disease activity—think of them as the undercover agents providing updates on what's happening inside. For example, fecal calprotectin levels above 100 µg/g after surgery suggest a recurrence of Crohn's with high sensitivity, making it a critical tool for postoperative monitoring.[14] We'll cover post-op IBD in later vignettes.

Although CRP is not exclusively specific to Crohn's inflammation, its levels can also be useful in monitoring the disease's progression and how well a patient responds to treatments, particularly infliximab. Speaking of which, starting with CRP levels above 15mg/L might hint at a bumpier road in responding to this treatment, but seeing those levels drop is a good sign that things are moving in the right direction.[15]

And then there's imaging, especially CTE and MRE, as was used in this case. These techniques are especially useful for examining small bowel disease and can be very helpful to examine areas beyond colonoscopy, but without requiring invasive enteroscopy. Moreover, improvements in MRE scores have been linked to clinical improvements, further validating their use in monitoring infliximab treatment.[16]

Small bowel ultrasound is also playing a larger role in the non-invasive monitoring of Crohn's disease, particularly valuable for its ability to visualize the small intestine. This technique is adept at identifying inflammation, complications such as strictures and fistulas, and monitoring disease progression over time.[17] Its advantages include the absence of radiation exposure, making it a safer option for repeated assessments, and its utility in guiding clinical decisions regarding therapy adjustments and interventions. Particularly popular in European healthcare settings (but quickly gaining traction in the U.S.), small bowel ultrasound complements other diagnostic tools by offering a detailed view of bowel wall thickness and other signs of disease activity, facilitating a comprehensive approach to managing Crohn's disease.

The pursuit of mucosal healing stands as a primary treatment objective, with endoscopy playing a pivotal role in assessing this goal. Mucosal healing, defined by the complete absence of ulceration, is a strong predictor of long-term remission and decreased need for surgical interventions.

Case 1.3: Flare Factors

A 35-year-old man with a history of Crohn's disease, previously in remission on infliximab to maintain remission, now presents with recurrent bloody diarrhea and worsening abdominal pain. The patient has experienced a recent upsurge in work-related stress and is a current smoker. Approximately one month prior, he sustained a sprained ankle during a basketball game in Bloomington, Indiana and has been using non-steroidal anti-inflammatory drugs (NSAIDs) for pain management since the injury. On top of that, he received clarithromycin from his primary care provider for a recent upper respiratory tract infection. Despite previous stability on infliximab, he is now presenting to your office for management of increasing flares

Know your guidelines!

What modifiable risk factors might be contributing to this clinical picture?

Case 1.3: What do the guidelines say?

Source: ACG 2018 Crohn's Disease Guidelines[1]

When a patient with IBD has a flare-up after being in remission, it's important to think about what might be triggering the problem. Could it be low adherence with treatments? A bacterial infection like *C. difficile*? Some kind of dietary indiscretion? New-onset small intestinal bacterial overgrowth (SIBO)? You need to Sherlock Holmes this situation, thinking carefully about all the clues and tracking down potential culprits.

In this case, there are several possible contributors to the flare-up. First, this patient has been using NSAIDs. These meds are known for their potential to exacerbate Crohn's symptoms.[18] Observational studies and clinical reports have revealed an association between NSAID use and IBD flare-ups.[19] There's enough evidence to suggest that steering clear of these meds is wise.

What about smoking? In Crohn's disease, it's a no-go. Smoking is like fuel to the fire for Crohn's and is associated with a higher need for surgeries, more hospital stays, and can even influence the disease to take on a more aggressive form.[20] Quitting smoking isn't just good advice for general health; for Crohn's patients, it can dial down disease flares and cut down the reliance on meds.

This patient also recently took antibiotics. It turns out that antibiotics are a bit of a mixed bag with Crohn's disease. They can disrupt the microbiome and may sometimes stir up IBD symptoms. On the other hand, one study pointed to antibiotics possibly reducing the risk of a flare,[21] but it's a complex picture, especially with the risk of infections like *C. difficile*. The effects of antibiotics on Crohn's disease aren't black and white and need careful consideration. That said, the ACG guidelines emphasize that if an IBD patient needs antibiotics, they should get their antibiotics. On average, the benefits will outweigh the risks. Just always be sure the antibiotics are warranted—just like with any other patient.

Lastly, the mental health angle—stress, depression, and anxiety aren't just tough on the mind; they can sometimes make Crohn's worse, too. [22] These aren't just feelings; they're factors that tangibly lower life quality and can make managing Crohn's harder, from adhering to treatment plans to the overall impact on health. Addressing these with as much care as the physical aspects of the disease is key to holistic care. For example, in Dr. Spiegel's lab at Cedars-Sinai, his team will sometimes use virtual reality (VR) therapy with IBD patients to help lower stress, ideally reducing stress hormones and possibly reducing immune-mediated inflammation (that's the hope anyway). Heck, this patient is likely a devout Indiana University basketball fan since he is from Bloomington, and it is quite stressful being an avid IU fan! So, whether it's stress from dealing with the disease itself or the added strain from depression, tackling these head-on can make a real difference in symptom management and overall well-being.

So, effective management of Crohn's disease is not just about the meds. Lifestyle factors like NSAID use, smoking, antibiotic effects, and even mental health play huge roles in either fueling the fire or dousing the flames. **Figure 1.2**, below, provide a mnemonic to help "trigger" your mind about IBD flare factors.

Figure 1.2. *A memory aid to learn the triggers of an IBD flare. They conveniently spell out the word "TRIGGER"*

Tobacco (smoking)
Rx non-adherence
Infections (especially *C. diff*)
Gut microbiota changes (e.g., antibiotics, SIBO)
Gastrointestinal irritants (e.g., NSAIDS)
Eating habits (diet and nutrition factors)
Restlessness (stress, both emotional and psychological)

Case 1.4: Flare Fundamentals

A 31-year-old individual presents with a 2-month history of recurrent abdominal pain, diarrhea, and recent onset of joint pain, primarily affecting the knees and ankles. The patient describes these symptoms as progressively worsening, leading to discomfort and having an impact on daily activities. Family history is notable for IBD in a first-degree relative.

Vital signs are normal, and body mass index (BMI) is 24 kg/m². There is right lower quadrant tenderness but no rebound or guarding. Rectal exam does not reveal evidence of perianal fistulae or blood. There are no skin rashes or eye findings.

Initial investigations, including blood tests, show elevated inflammatory markers. Stool studies are negative for infectious causes, including *C. difficile* and other common enteric pathogens. Imaging with MRE reveals inflammation and edema localized to the terminal ileum, consistent with ileitis. Colonoscopy with biopsies confirms granulomatous inflammation. Serologic markers further support the diagnosis of Crohn's disease, and other potential mimics of the condition, such as tuberculosis and sarcoidosis, have been ruled out.

Know your guidelines!

How would you treat this patient next?

Case 1.4: What do the guidelines say?

Source: ACG 2018 Crohn's Disease Guidelines[1]

This patient has mild-to-moderate Crohn's disease and needs treatment. It might be tempting to reach for prednisone right out the gate, but the ACG guidelines indicate that steroids are primarily used for people with moderate-to-severe disease activity, which isn't quite the case here. Instead, it is better to use a more directed, less systemic treatment first line, unless symptoms become more aggressive. Also, this patient does not yet have predictors of severe disease, such as early age of diagnosis, elevated BMI, fistulizing or stenotic disease, or extensive bowel involvement. That may all occur in time, but as of now, a "top down" approach of using big guns like an upfront biologic seems unnecessary.

While it may not always pack the same punch as traditional oral corticosteroids, controlled ileal-release (CIR) **budesonide** at a dose of 9 mg daily stands out as a solid option for easing symptoms in the short term for patients with mild-to-moderate Crohn's disease localized to the terminal ileum and right colon.[23] CIR budesonide, designed to release specifically in the pH environment of the ileum, offers both high local effectiveness and minimal systemic absorption—roughly 10%–20%. This formulation's targeted release and first-pass metabolism significantly limit whole-body corticosteroid effects, making it a compelling choice for active ileocecal Crohn's management, as supported by randomized, placebo-controlled trials. This strategic balance of localized action versus systemic exposure underpins the appeal of CIR budesonide for this specific Crohn's disease presentation. Just bear in mind that budesonide should not be used indefinitely. The ACG guidelines recommend only using for four months, at which time a steroid-sparing agent, such as azathioprine (AZA), 6-mercaptopurine (6-MP), methotrexate (MTX), or most commonly, a biologic, should be considered. We'll discuss more about these in future vignettes.

What about **mesalamine**? Should this agent be used as first-line therapy for patients with ileal Crohn's? Recall that mesalamine is 5-aminosalicylic acid (5-ASA), whereas **sulfasalazine** combines 5-ASA with sulfapyridine, a sulfa moiety that helps transport 5-ASA to the colon. The story is slightly different between using mesalamine vs sulfasalazine in the management of Crohn's disease, and truth be told, neither is much good for Crohn's (in contrast to UC, as we'll see later). Studies evaluating oral mesalamine for active Crohn's have not consistently shown it to be more effective than a placebo for inducing remission or promoting mucosal healing.[24] In contrast, sulfasalazine has shown some efficacy at doses of 3–6 g daily for treating symptoms in patients with mild-to-moderately active colonic Crohn's or ileo-colonic CD, but its benefits don't extend to isolated small bowel disease. Moreover, sulfasalazine hasn't

outperformed placebo in achieving mucosal healing in Crohn's, so it's really not a top choice (yet, we still see a fair amount of 5-ASA use in Crohn's disease). While 5-ASA suppositories and enemas are effective for managing rectal and sigmoid disease in UC, their utility in Crohn's, especially as topical mesalamine, offers limited advantage and these medications are not useful for managing this patient with isolated small bowel disease.

Is there a role for antibiotics? In the past, **metronidazole** or **ciprofloxacin** were often used to help induce remission for active Crohn's on the theory that chronic intestinal inflammation stems, in part, from an abnormal immune reaction to the gut's flora in those who are genetically susceptible. However, the ACG guidelines are less enthusiastic about using antibiotics. Studies have shown neither metronidazole nor ciprofloxacin outperform placebo in remission induction.[25] These medications also haven't proven effective in mucosal healing for active luminal Crohn's. Broad-spectrum antibiotics, though, are still warranted for addressing pyogenic complications like abscesses, but that's not relevant in this vignette.

Postoperative recurrence prevention is one area where metronidazole shows promise, especially when used alongside AZA. Ornidazole has also demonstrated effectiveness in preventing post-surgical recurrence, both clinically and endoscopically.[26] Rifaximin, particularly a novel enteric form, shows potential benefits for mild-to-moderate Crohn's, but it's still not commonly used for this indication.[27]

Related, exploration into the role of mycobacterial infections in CD development has concluded that, due to the absence of mycobacteria in tissues and the lack of patient improvement with anti-mycobacterial regimens, these therapies are also not recommended for active Crohn's disease management, nor for induction or maintenance of remission.[28]

Finally, what about the **role of diet** for managing Crohn's disease? The ACG guidelines are not too bullish. Although dietary interventions, including elemental, semi-elemental, and specific defined diets, such as the Mediterranean diet,[29] have shown some promise in reducing mucosal inflammation markers and improving symptoms in Crohn's, their benefits tend to be temporary, with a return to normal eating often leading to a resurgence of symptoms and inflammation. As such, these dietary strategies might best serve as complementary to conventional therapies during the induction phase for certain patients, particularly those at a lower risk for aggressive disease progression. That said, there's a lot of room still for high-quality, carefully conducted diet studies across all of gastroenterology, including IBD, and it stands to reason that what we put into our gut will obviously affect how it operates and, consequently, our overall health. Afterall, it was Hippocrates who said, "all disease begins in the gut." We eagerly await more data on dietary interventions for IBD.

Case 1.5: Crohn's in Crescendo

A 37-year-old patient presents with a 3-week history of worsening abdominal pain, diarrhea (approximately 6 episodes per day, occasionally bloody), and a significant weight loss of 8 lbs. The patient reports a past medical history of Crohn's disease diagnosed 5 years ago, predominantly affecting the ileum and colon, with a previous good response to maintenance therapy with 6-MP until this recent flare.

On physical exam, the patient appears fatigued and moderately dehydrated. Abdominal palpation reveals tenderness in the right lower quadrant without peritoneal signs. There's no palpable mass, but the patient expresses discomfort during palpation. No extraintestinal manifestations such as joint swelling or skin lesions are noted.

Labs show elevated inflammatory markers (CRP and ESR) with anemia (hemoglobin [Hgb] 10.2 g/dL), and a slight increase in white blood cell count. Stool cultures and tests for *C. difficile* toxin are negative. Fecal calprotectin levels are markedly elevated.

Abdominal imaging, including an MRE, reveals thickening of the terminal ileum with enhanced mucosal contrast uptake. There are no signs of fistulae, abscesses, or strictures.

Know your guidelines!

How would you treat this patient next?

Case 1.5: What do the guidelines say?

Source: ACG 2018 Crohn's Disease Guidelines[1]

This patient has moderate-to-severe Crohn's disease and needs timely systemic therapy to avoid further complications and worse outcomes. Often, a patient like this will receive a course of high-dose oral or intravenous corticosteroids to induce remission, followed by a longer-term plan for maintenance therapy. So, let's start with reviewing what the guidelines say about steroids, then we'll look at some of the other key treatments, including biologics, that may be warranted for managing this patient.

Corticosteroids. Oral corticosteroids like prednisone or methyl-prednisolone, and in more severe cases, intravenous forms, are typically effective for quick symptom relief during flares. However, we all know that these meds can cause too many side effects, including bone loss, mood changes, sleep issues, high blood pressure, and more, making them a suboptimal therapy for long-term management. That said, the usual starting dose for a limited treatment course ranges from 40 to 60 mg/day of prednisone, with some cases requiring up to 1 mg/kg body weight per day. The initial dose is generally kept for 1-2 weeks before gradually tapering down. The tapering should not extend beyond 3 months, and doses above 60 mg/day are not advised due to lack of evidence and potential for increased side effects.

Despite their effectiveness in symptom management, corticosteroids don't necessarily promote mucosal healing and carry risks like dependency, refractoriness, and even leading to complications like abscesses and fistulas. Given these limitations, corticosteroids are recommended for short-term use only and should be phased out in favor of steroid-sparing agents like biologics, AZA, or 6-MP. As an aside, it's still surprising to see patients come to us on long-term steroids, having never been tapered off these agents. Remember, it's simply unacceptable this far into the 21st century to keep IBD patients on long-term steroids. We have too many other therapies available for that. Even AI knows steroids are bad. Let's do better than AI!

Immunomodulators. For those cases of moderate-to-severe Crohn's where corticosteroids just aren't cutting it, the guidelines indicate that thiopurines like AZA and 6-MP can be used for a steroid-sparing strategy (although biologics tend to be used more commonly these days, more on that soon). Thiopurines work well for keeping the disease in check over the long haul rather than quick symptom relief, taking about 8 to 12 weeks to kick in. MTX also gets a nod from the ACG guidelines, especially for steroid-dependent or resistant Crohn's, but comes with a caution for reproductive health. Men and women need to use effective birth control during and a bit after treatment due to potential risks to fertility and pregnancy. Long-term MTX use also carries a small risk for progressive fibrotic liver disease leading to portal hypertension and cirrhosis. So, you gotta be careful with MTX and monitor while using it.

Dosing is key with immunomodulators: AZA up to 2.5 mg/kg/day, 6-MP up to 1.5 mg/kg/day, or methotrexate 15–25 mg/week, and they can also work well in combination with biologics to reduce anti-drug antibody formation.

As for cyclosporine, tacrolimus, and mycophenolate mofetil, they haven't shown much promise for tackling active luminal CD, so they're usually not part of the playbook.

Biologics. Okay, this is a very big topic, so we'll focus on the highlights here, and continue to cover some of the finer points in forthcoming vignettes.

Anti-TNFα Agents. These include infliximab, adalimumab, and certolizumab pegol. Golimumab is another biologic in this class but it's currently only recommended for use in UC. In short, the ACG guidelines strongly recommend use of anti-TNFα agents for managing mild-to-severe Crohn's disease, particularly cases that are resistant to treatment with corticosteroids. Combining an anti-TNF with an immunomodulator is more effective than using either treatment alone, revealing a synergistic benefit of combination therapy.[30] Also, using these treatments earlier in the course of the disease, particularly within the first 2 years of diagnosis, is associated with better outcomes compared to later use of anti-TNFs. Here are some key points to remember when prescribing an anti-TNF therapy:

- Before starting these meds, be sure **to rule out latent tuberculosis** (TB). If positive, the patient must receive treatment for TB prior to starting a biologic, preferably several weeks to months in advance.

- Also **screen for hepatitis B** virus infection, which could reactivate upon starting a biologic. If the patient is seronegative for hepatitis B, then they need to be vaccinated before starting therapy. If positive for hep B surface antigen (sAg), then begin antiviral agents before starting the anti-TNF. Do you also need to check for hepatitis C virus (HCV)? Yes, even though HCV doesn't reactivate with biologics, there could be progression of liver disease in those with advanced fibrosis. Thus, your authors would start the short oral course of antiviral therapy (which has a 98% cure rate), before starting anti-TNF therapy if possible.

- **Vaccinate** for pneumococcus, herpes zoster, human papilloma virus, influenza, and hepatitis A, ideally before starting biologics.

- Smokers should be informed that they are less likely to respond to therapy if they continue smoking, and should **strongly consider quitting.**

- These agents harbor a **small risk of lymphoma**. About 6 per 10,000 patient-years using an anti-TNF may develop lymphoma, whereas background rates in the general population around 2 per 10,000 patient-years of follow-up.

- The guidelines emphasize that **biosimilars** available for infliximab and adalimumab are non-inferior to traditional anti-TNFs and can be used for both induction and maintenance of Crohn's disease.

Anti-a4 Integrin Antibodies. These agents, including natalizumab and vedolizumab, inhibit leukocyte trafficking and can be highly effective for both induction and maintenance therapy of moderate-to-severe IBD. However, natalizumab can trigger the dreaded progressive multifocal leukoencephalopathy (PML), a rare and devastating neurological condition caused by the John Cunningham virus (JCV) that affects 1 in 100 patients testing positive for the JCV antibody. Thus, if you ever consider using natalizumab (which is very rare these days), then it's vital to first screen for JCV antibody and confirm negativity. Additionally, if JCV antibody is initially negative, then continual monitoring for JCV antibody while on natalizumab therapy is required. Thankfully, vedolizumab, the other anti-integrin therapy, has not been linked to PML outside of one case in a patient who had concurrent HIV—a known risk factor for PML. This benefit is thought to result from vedolizumab's greater specificity for the gut, rather than affecting leukocyte trafficking systemically. There are few head-to-head studies comparing these drugs vs anti-TNF agents, but a network meta-analysis suggests that adalimumab or combo therapy with infliximab and AZA is more effective than vedolizumab.[31]

Anti IL-12/23 Agents. Ustekinumab, targeting IL-12 and IL-23 through anti-p40 antibodies, steps up as a viable option for Crohn's disease patients who haven't found success with the usual treatments—think steroids, immunomodulators, and anti-TNF therapies. It's like bringing in a new, specialized player off the bench after the standard lineup hasn't quite sealed the deal. Its safety profile is particularly noteworthy, having established a solid track record in treating psoriasis without significantly raising the risks of serious infections or cancer. Finally, risankizumab has also recently gained regulatory approval for Crohn's disease treatment. This agent targets the P-19 component and inhibits IL-23.

Case 1.6: Infliximab's Fading Force

A 43-year-old man with Crohn's disease, who had shown improvement on infliximab at a dose of 5 mg/kg, is experiencing a flare-up of symptoms 5 weeks following his most recent infusion. Despite his initial positive response, recent endoscopic evaluation demonstrates ongoing inflammation, and tests for enteric pathogens have returned negative results. Laboratory analysis reveals undetectable trough levels of infliximab, with no antibodies detected against the drug.

Know your guidelines!

1. What is the most likely explanation for this situation?

2. How should you manage this case next?

Case 1.6: What do the guidelines say?

Source: ACG 2018 Crohn's Disease Guidelines[1]

In situations where a patient previously responsive to infliximab begins to show reduced effectiveness, it's crucial to first rule out alternative causes for the symptom resurgence. In an earlier vignette, we discussed the "TRIGGER"s for IBD flares, and those must be considered here, too.

But this situation requires us to understand why some people might lose responsiveness to infliximab or other biologics, and to distinguish between "secondary non-responders," who initially benefit from infliximab but later lose response, and "primary non-responders" who derive no initial benefit.

If no alternative explanation emerges for worsening symptoms, the next step involves assessing both anti-drug antibodies and infliximab trough levels prior to the upcoming dose. The absence of antibodies to infliximab (ATI) alongside undetectable trough levels of the drug suggests that the issue may not be immunogenicity but rather an inadequate dosage of biologic.

Given these findings, the patient's infliximab regimen should be reassessed. An increase in the infliximab dosage, potentially up to 10 mg/kg from the initial 5 mg/kg, alongside consideration for more frequent administration, may be warranted to regain control over the disease activity. This approach allows for the continuation of infliximab treatment under a revised dosing strategy, provided the patient tolerates the medication well, before contemplating the transition to alternative therapies or discontinuation of infliximab.

Case 1.7: Present, But Not Accounted For

A 29-year-old woman with a history of Crohn's disease, previously well-controlled on infliximab 5 mg/kg, presents with a recurrence of symptoms including abdominal pain and diarrhea 8 weeks after her last infusion. Despite her prior good response to therapy, she now reports a noticeable decline in symptom control.

Extensive workup to identify potential triggers of this flare has been undertaken, including studies for pathogens like *C. difficile* and mucosal biopsies for cytomegalovirus (CMV), all of which returned negative. The patient does not report recent use of NSAIDs, has not been prescribed antibiotics in the past 6 months, and there are no dietary changes or new stressors reported. Laboratory investigations reveal detectable infliximab trough levels. Additionally, testing for antibodies to infliximab is negative.

Know your guidelines!

1. What is the most likely explanation for this situation?

2. How should you manage this case next?

Case 1.7: What do the guidelines say?

Source: ACG 2018 Crohn's Disease Guidelines[1]

Here's another situation where a patient initially responding to a biologic gets worse. Once again, it's important to consider the "TRIGGER" factors and rule-out a modifiable reason for the flare. In this case, there are important clues in the therapeutic drug monitoring results. In particular, there is a measurable infliximab drug level, but no evidence of anti-drug antibodies.

Since there are no antibodies to infliximab, this isn't a problem with immunogenicity. The drug levels are measurable, meaning the biologic is not being cleared out by the immune system. Instead, the issue here is "mechanistic escape," where the patient is just not responding to the medicine anymore. It's like the drug is "present, but not accounted for," because the body is essentially ignoring it's presence.

In this situation, not only does infliximab need to be stopped, but no other anti-TNFα therapy should be used. For example, rather than switching to adalimumab or certolizumab-pegol, which share the same anti-TNFα mechanism, it's more appropriate to try another mechanism of action. Other options might include anti-IL12/23 therapy or anti-integrin therapy.

Case 1.8: A Stalled Start

A 40-year-old woman with a recent diagnosis of moderate-to-severe Crohn's disease presents with persistent symptoms despite standard treatment. Prior to initiating biological therapy, she reported significant abdominal pain, frequent diarrhea, and had experienced a weight loss of 10 lbs over 2 months. The decision to start infliximab was made after conventional therapies, including corticosteroids and aminosalicylates, failed to achieve symptom control, and imaging studies confirmed active inflammation in the terminal ileum.

The patient received infliximab 5 mg/kg infusions at weeks 0, 2, and 6 as part of the induction therapy. Despite this regimen, she reports no improvement in her symptoms; abdominal pain and diarrhea persist, and there's been no weight recovery. Laboratory tests continue to show elevated inflammatory markers, and a follow-up endoscopic assessment reveals ongoing mucosal inflammation in the ileum, without significant change from her pre-treatment evaluation.

Know your guidelines!

1. What is the most likely explanation for this situation?
2. How should you manage this case next?

Case 1.8: What do the guidelines say?

Source: ACG 2018 Crohn's Disease Guidelines[1]

This case exemplifies a primary nonresponse scenario. Despite completing a standard course of infliximab treatment, the patient experienced no therapeutic benefits. This differs from secondary non-responders, who initially respond to therapy but subsequently experience a loss of efficacy. Given the lack of response from the outset, pursuing further treatment with infliximab or similar anti-TNFα agents is not advisable. Alternative therapeutic strategies should be explored, including anti-IL12/23 therapy or anti-integrin therapy. Surgical interventions may also be considered, as we will discuss in future vignettes.

Case 1.9: Finding a Fistula

A 38-year-old patient with a known history of Crohn's disease presents with new-onset anal pain and noticeable discharge, symptoms that have progressively worsened over the past few weeks. The patient reports no recent changes in diet, medication, or overall health status that could otherwise explain these symptoms.

During the consultation, the patient mentions that the pain intensifies during bowel movements and sitting, significantly impacting daily activities and quality of life.

On exam, there is localized swelling and redness around the anal area, with a visible draining fistula near the anal opening.

Know your guidelines!

1. What diagnostic testing is indicated?

2. How will the results of testing determine your treatment plan?

Case 1.9: What do the guidelines say?

Source: ACG 2018 Crohn's Disease Guidelines

Perianal fistulas in Crohn's disease represent a complex and challenging complication, marked by abnormal connections between the epithelialized surface of the anal canal and the perianal skin. These fistulas arise when inflammation that characteristically penetrates the intestinal wall in Crohn's disease extends to involve the anal and rectal areas, often creating a tract or channel. This inflammatory process may begin as a simple perianal abscess and subsequently burrow its way to the surface, forming a fistulous tract (**Figure 1.3**).

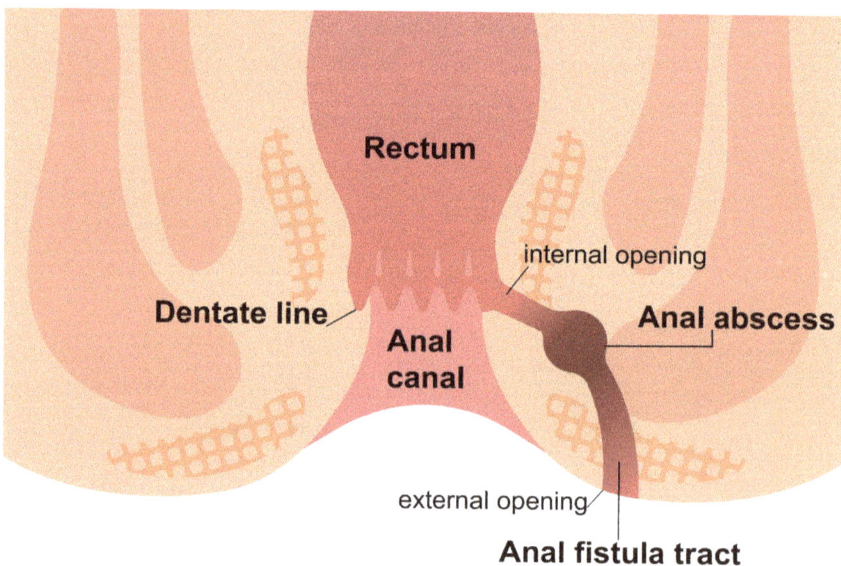

Figure 1.3. *Cross-section depiction of an anal fistula tract with an abscess.*

Anatomically, perianal fistulas can be classified based on their relationship to the structures of the anal sphincter. According to the Parks classification, fistulas are categorized as intersphincteric, transsphincteric, suprasphincteric, and extrasphincteric.[32] That's a lot of sphincterics*! The most common types among Crohn's

*We kind of wish that were a real word**

    ** We sometimes like to use footnotes.

patients are the intersphincteric and transsphincteric fistulas. The intersphincteric fistula, which runs between the internal and external anal sphincters, often results in fewer symptoms and is often simpler to treat. On the other hand, transsphincteric fistulas, which penetrate both sphincters and extend to the ischiorectal fossa, pose greater therapeutic challenges and have a higher risk of recurrence and incontinence. **Figure 1.4** breaks down the different types of fistulas.

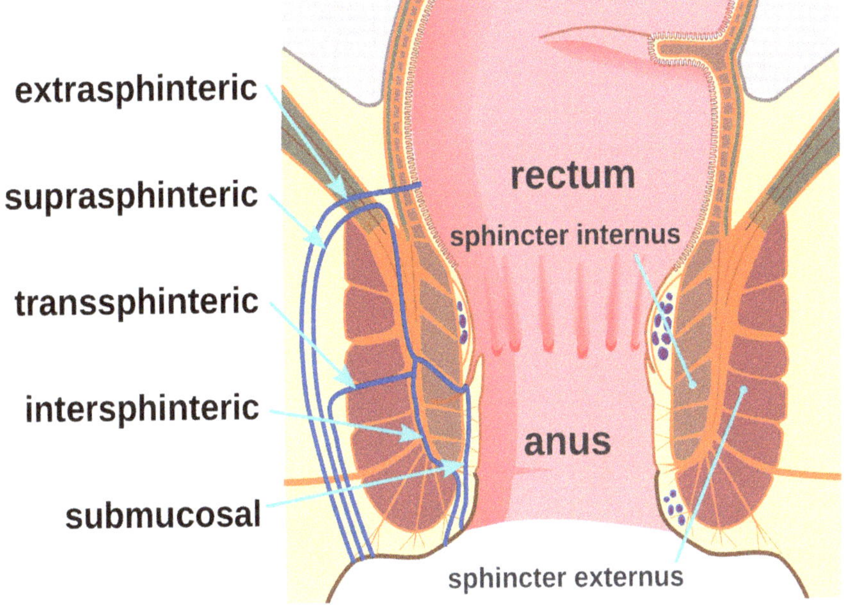

Figure 1.4. *Parks Classification of perianal fistulas.*

Perianal fistulizing disease occurs in about one-third of patients with Crohn's disease at some point in their disease course. These fistulas are not only painful and distressing but can also be resistant to treatment, reflecting the aggressive nature of penetrating Crohn's disease. The prevalence and recurrence of these conditions emphasize the importance of a comprehensive management strategy that incorporates both medical and surgical interventions tailored to the

About one-third of patients with Crohn's develop a perianal fistula

type and complexity of the fistula and the overall condition of the patient.

When dealing with a case like this, where perianal symptoms suggest fistulizing disease, the guidelines point us toward a few key diagnostic steps. First off, you should consider performing an MRI of the pelvis, which is the go-to imaging to map out the anatomy of fistulas. This test helps to see the extent of the problem and determine whether there's any hidden mischief like abscesses that need attention.

Also, be sure to perform a thorough rectal examination, potentially under anesthesia with colorectal surgery if needed, which gives a clearer view and understanding of the fistula's trajectory and involvement. Lab work is a given to check for signs of infection and to get a sense of the overall inflammatory activity, so we're talking CRP, ESR, and a complete blood count.

If the MRI shows a simple fistula without any complications, you might manage it with medication alone—think antibiotics or biologics like infliximab or adalimumab. More on that in a moment. But, if the patient has a complex network or abscesses, then surgery might be necessary to drain the abscesses and possibly place a seton to keep things under control. Let's break down the options, approaching three categories: simple fistulas (i.e., distal to dentate line, single tract), complex fistulas, (i.e., above dentate line and/or branching tracts) and internal fistulas (i.e., non-draining to skin). Here are key bullet points from the ACG guidelines:

Simple Fistula Management

- *Observation.* Small abscesses (<5 mm) often do not require intervention. Asymptomatic simple fistulas often need no treatment but should be carefully monitored.

- *Antibiotic considerations.* For superficial and simple fistulas that minimally involve sphincter muscles, antibiotics like metronidazole or ciprofloxacin can be effective. They're typically used for 4 to 8 weeks to treat both the fistula and any associated mucosal disease.

- ***Interventional Techniques.*** Symptomatic simple fistulas can be managed with non-cutting setons or fistulotomy if the fistula is low risk for causing incontinence, typically when they do not extensively involve sphincter muscles.

Complex Fistula Management

- ***Initial Approach***. Complex fistulas, characterized by their involvement across sphincters or having multiple tracts, require more aggressive management. Seton placement is commonly employed to facilitate drainage and prevent abscess formation.

- ***Medical Therapy***. Concurrent with surgical intervention, medical therapies such as anti-TNF agents are recommended. These help reduce inflammation and close fistula tracts over time. While antibiotics can be effective in reducing symptoms and possibly healing simple fistulas, they're less effective for complex perianal fistulas but may still alleviate symptoms. While not a replacement for surgical drainage in cases of abscesses, antibiotics can serve as an adjunct to manage perianal sepsis. Also, keep in mind that combining anti-TNF agents with antibiotics has demonstrated greater efficacy than monotherapy in reducing fistula drainage and improving outcomes.

- ***Surgical Considerations***. In refractory cases, more invasive surgeries like diverting ostomy may be necessary to allow the inflamed tissues to heal. Ultimately, for non-responsive and severe cases, proctectomy or total proctocolectomy with permanent stoma might be indicated.

Management of Internal Fistulas

Rectovaginal Fistulas. Treatment typically starts with medical management using anti-TNF therapy with or without immuno-modulators to reduce inflammation. Surgical intervention may include fistula excision followed by the placement of a mucosal advancement flap to promote healing.

Enterovesical Fistulas. These are managed based on symptomatology; recurrent urinary infections may require bowel resection and bladder repair. Medical therapy aims to reduce inflammation before surgery.

Treatment Strategy. For all internal fistulas, ensuring the absence of active infection and inflammation before surgery is crucial to improve surgical outcomes.

Considerations for Severe Cases

Diverting Ostomy. In cases with extensive perianal damage or severe inflammation, temporary diversion of the fecal stream via ostomy can help heal the affected areas.

Proctectomy. Reserved as a last resort, this surgery involves the complete removal of the rectum and is considered for patients with persistent, debilitating symptoms and significant quality of life impairment.

This array of medical and surgical approaches underscores the importance of a tailored treatment approach based on the complexity of the fistu-la and the individual patient's overall health and response to past treatments.

Case 1.10: Smoke Signals

A 42-year-old man diagnosed 6 months ago with ileocolonic Crohn's disease managed on biologics recently underwent surgical resection of 150 cm of the terminal ileum due to active and fistulizing disease despite therapy—his first surgery for IBD. During the procedure, a fistulectomy was also performed due to the presence of an internal fistula. Notably, the patient is a current smoker and occasionally uses NSAIDs for joint pain. He is now three weeks out from surgery and his postoperative course has been uneventful so far.

Know your guidelines!

1. What risk factors does this patient have for postoperative recurrence?

2. What treatments are warranted at this time?

Case 1.10: What do the guidelines say?

Source: ACG 2018 Crohn's Disease Guidelines[1]

Despite our best medical efforts to control IBD, medications often fall short, mandating surgical intervention. Approximately 80% of patients with Crohn's disease will require some form of gastrointestinal surgery. That's a lot, so it's crucial to understand how best to manage post-operative patients. This involves recognizing risk factors that can influence their disease course after surgery, which is the focus of this case.

So, what are the risk factors for post-op recurrence? The title of this vignette should give you a hint: smoking! It is critical that patients stop smoking, if at all possible, because that's the #1 predictor of post-operative recurrence.[33] Another risk seen here is penetrating disease, which also portends a worse post-operative prognosis. Additionally, progression to surgery despite treatment with immunomodulators or biologic agents often indicates an aggressive disease phenotype, suggesting a higher recurrence risk. Other factors include a short interval between diagnosis and surgery, disease affecting both the ileum and colon, and use of NSAIDs. Again, all seen here. Then there are other risk factors not evident in in this case, including presence of perianal fistula, extensive bowel resection, and pre-surgery corticosteroid use. **Table 1.3** lists these risk factors:

> Active smoking is the #1 predictor of post-operative recurrence in Crohn's disease

Because this patient is at high risk for recurrence, it's important to stay aggressive with post-op therapy. The ACG guidelines recommend using anti-TNF therapy in this situation because these agents may alter the natural history of disease after surgery. This is supported by a meta-analysis data bolstering the case for anti-TNFs, showing they substantially reduce both clinical and endoscopic recurrence when compared to placebo.[34] A recent network meta-analysis compared the efficacy of

> Use anti-TNF after surgery in those at high-risk for recurrence

ustekinumab, vedolizumab, and 2 anti-TNF therapies (infliximab and adalimumab) for the prevention of postoperative Crohn's disease recurrence and found them to be equally efficacious.[35]

Table 1.3. *Risk factors for post-operative recurrence of Crohn's disease.*

Smoking
Penetrating / fistulizing disease
Progression to surgery despite immunomodulators or biologics
Short interval between diagnosis and surgery
Disease affecting both ileum and colon
Use of NSAIDs
Extensive bowel resection
Pre-surgery corticosteroid use

For patients at low risk of postoperative Crohn's disease recurrence—those who are nonsmokers without penetrating disease and no prior surgeries—the guidelines suggest a wait-and-see approach involving a colonoscopy at 6 months to check for recurrence. If patients are nonsmokers but have penetrating disease and have not undergone surgery previously nor received any treatment, starting them on thiopurines, possibly along with metronidazole, makes sense. A follow-up colonoscopy at 6 months will help decide if biologic therapy needs to be added depending on the disease findings. For those with a history of resection within the last decade, proactive treatment with anti-TNF, optionally combined with an immunomodulator, is advisable. Alternatively, monotherapy with vedolizumab or ustekinumab may be used. A colonoscopy at 6 months post-surgery can provide further guidance on the treatment effectiveness and need for adjustments.

Case 1.11: UC Basics

A 30-year-old man presents with a 3-week history of experiencing fewer than 4 loose stools per day, occasionally noticing a trace of blood. He describes the urgency as mild and infrequent, with discomfort localized to the lower abdomen that is not significantly impacting his daily activities. Routine blood tests indicate normal hemoglobin levels, and inflammatory markers such as ESR and CRP are within normal limits. Fecal calprotectin is slightly elevated, between 150-200 µg/g. Albumin is normal. Stool studies do not reveal any evidence of infections. A diagnostic colonoscopy is performed, revealing mild erythema and decreased vascular pattern, extension continuously through the left colon, with a Mayo score of 1. Biopsies confirm evidence of architectural distortion with crypt abscesses, confirming the clinical suspicion of UC.

Know your guidelines!

1. How would you rate the disease severity of this case?

2. What does a Mayo score of 1 mean?

3. How would you judge this patient's overall prognosis based on the data presented so far?

4. How would you treat this patient?

Case 1.11: What do the guidelines say?

Source: ACG 2019 Ulcerative Colitis Guidelines[36]

This patient's UC can be classified as "mild." The ACG criteria for mild UC, as shown in **Table 1.4**, include having fewer than four stools per day with or without blood, no signs of systemic toxicity, and normal or mild elevation in inflammatory markers such as ESR or CRP. This patient's symptoms fit within these parameters. In contrast, more severe cases would be characterized by >6 bowel movements per day, continuous blood in stools, urgency, and possibly systemic signs like a high fever or elevated ESR and CRP levels beyond mild elevations, leading to different management strategies. In this case, the absence of these more severe signs and symptoms helps categorize the condition as mild.

Table 1.4. *American College of Gastroenterology Ulcerative Colitis Activity Index*[36]

	Remission	Mild	Moderate-Severe	Fulminant
Stools (#/d)	Formed stools	<4	>6	>10
Blood in stool	None	Intermittent	Frequent	Continuous
Urgency	None	Mild, occasional	Often	Continuous
Hemoglobin	Normal	Normal	<75% of normal	Transfusion required
ESR	<30	<30	>30	>30
CRP (mg/L)	Normal	Elevated	Elevated	Elevated
FC (μ/g)	<150-200	>150-200	>150-200	>150-200
Endoscopy (Mayo subscore)	0-1	1	2-3	3
UCEIS	0-1	2-4	5-8	7-8

The above factors are general guides for disease activity. With the exception of remission, a patient does not need to have all the factors to be considered in a specific category.
CRP, C-reactive protein; ESR, erythrocyte sedimentation rate; FC, fecal calprotectin; UCEIS, Ulcerative Colitis Endoscopic Index of Severity

The Mayo score, used for evaluating the severity of UC, ranges from 0 to 12 and is based on clinical findings, endoscopic findings, and a physician's global assessment.[37] A Mayo score of 1 is indicative of mild disease. It refers to the endoscopic sub-score, which assesses the appearance of the colonic mucosa during an endoscopy. A sub-score of 1 means there is mild inflammation characterized by erythema, decreased vascular pattern, and no friability. This scoring system helps clinicians to classify the severity of the disease, guide treatment decisions, and monitor the response to therapy.

The Mayo score levels are shown in **Figure 1.5**. A Mayo score of 1 is depicted by images showing mild changes in the colon. In contrast, a Mayo score of 2 is marked by more severe signs, including significant erythema, absence of the vascular pattern, friability, and the presence of erosions. A score of 3 indicates severe disease with features like spontaneous bleeding and ulceration of the colon. Each ascending score reflects an increase in the severity of disease, indicating more aggressive activity and typically correlating with more intense symptoms greater likelihood of hospitalization and surgery. By the way, the pictures in Figure 1.5 are all courtesy of the one-and-only Dr. David Rubin, of the University of Chicago, who provided the figure and led the ACG UC Guidelines. Dr. Rubin is a doctor of doctors, a fountain of wisdom, and someone worth reading, because his contributions to the field are enormous. Let's just say we're fans!

Based on the data presented so far, this patient does not yet exhibit poor prognosis factors for UC disease severity. **Figure 1.6.** provides a mnemonic to help remember the independent risk factors for poor prognosis ("ESCAPE UC").* Of the risk factors, this patient only has 1: diagnosis before age of 40.

*We love a good mnemonic! And we love a good footnote. Which this may, or may not be. Sorry to be a distraction. Guess we got distracted while writing. Okay, back to writing.

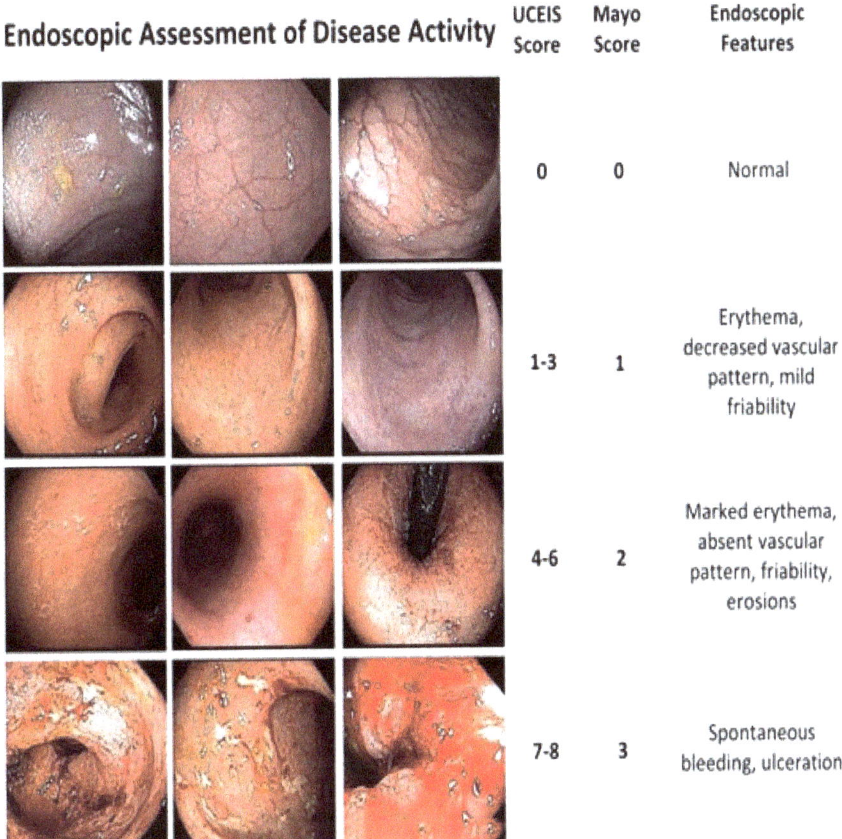

Figure 1.5. *Endoscopic images of UC patients with Mayo endoscopic sub-scores* [36]

Extensive colitis

Severe endoscopic disease (Mayo 3)

CRP elevated

Age <40 at diagnosis

Protein low (low serum albumin)

Emergencies (i.e., hospitalizations for UC)

UC (reminding us that these factors are specific to UC)

Figure 1.6. *Risk factors for poor UC prognosis (spells ESCAPE UC)*

Okay, how best to treat? This is mild UC, so we should start low, not go straight to big guns like biologics. This is a perfect case for using a 5-ASA as the frontline option. 5-ASA has been shown to be significantly more effective than placebo for inducing remission in UC (but remember, it does not work for Crohn's). For instance, the ACG guidelines highlight one meta-analysis covering 11 randomized controlled trials showing that 5-ASA treatments led to a substantial reduction in remission failure compared to placebo, emphasizing a robust effect irrespective of whether remission was evaluated through clinical symptoms or endoscopic appearance.[38]

Particularly for proctitis or left-sided UC, rectal formulations of 5-ASA have proven superior to placebo and even outperform rectal corticosteroids for inducing symptomatic remission.[39] The efficacy remains consistent across different dosages and formulations of 5-ASA, making it versatile for various extents of disease involvement. Although this patient does not have severe bouts of fecal urgency, when present, you should definitely think about using rectal 5-ASA as this approach has demonstrated superiority over steroid enemas. It's often the proctitis that most impacts quality of life, even more than the colitis. When the rectal inflammation is doused, patients typically feel way better, faster, even if the rest of the colon still needs to heal.

In cases where disease activity extends beyond the rectum, combination therapies is superior to monotherapy for symptom control. Adding rectal enemas to oral 5-ASAs (at least 2 g/day) significantly enhances remission induction over oral therapy alone.[40] Meanwhile, for more extensive colitis, higher doses of oral 5-ASA (e.g., 4.8 g/day) may be necessary.

If 5-ASA fails, the next step might involve corticosteroids to induce remission. Budesonide, particularly the MMX formulation at 9 mg/day, is preferred for its local effect and minimal systemic absorption, shown to be effective in achieving clinical and endo-scopic remission.

Lastly, while use of probiotics like VSL#3® and *Escherichia coli* Nissle 1917 has been explored, the evidence remains inconclusive and generally not recommended for routine use. Fecal microbio-ta transplant (FMT) has shown promise in some trials but is not standard treatment due to variable outcomes and lack of signifi-cant steroid-sparing effect. We'll come back to FMT in Chapter 2 when we discuss *C. difficile* treatment.

Case 1.12: Urgent UC

A 35-year-old woman with a previously diagnosed UC extending to the splenic flexure is now experiencing a significant flare. Previously well-controlled on oral mesalamine, she has seen an increase in symptoms over the past few weeks. She reports up to 8 bloody, loose stools per day along with abdominal pain, fecal urgency, and troublesome fatigue, all impacting her daily activities. Although her appetite is diminished, she is able to eat and keep food down.

She does not report recent travel, new dietary changes, or antibiotic use. Infectious causes, including *C. difficile*, have been excluded through stool studies. Vital signs are normal, and exam does not reveal an acute abdomen. Laboratory tests show a CRP level of 35 mg/L and an ESR of 50 mm/hr. Her hemoglobin is decreased to 10.2 g/dL, and fecal calprotectin is significantly elevated at 500 µg/g.

A colonoscopy reveals extensive ulcerative inflammation with erosions from the rectum to the splenic flexure, consistent with a Mayo endoscopic sub-score of 3. Biopsies confirm active colitis without signs of dysplasia.

Know your guidelines!

1. How would you rate the disease severity of this case?

2. Should this patient be admitted to the hospital?

3. How would you treat this patient?

Case 1.12: What do the guielines say?

Source: ACG 2019 Ulcerative Colitis Guidelines[36]

This patient is getting pretty sick. You need to act definitively to cool down the colon before things get worse. We can classify this case as a moderate-to-severe flare based upon the ACG UC Activity Index previously shown in **Table 1.4**. There are over six bowel movements per day, all bloody, along with fecal urgency, anemia, elevated inflammatory markers (ESR >30 and CRP elevated), and a very high fecal calprotectin that's well above the 150-200 level characterizing severe inflammation. The Mayo endoscopic sub-score is maxed out at 3, rounding out the picture of a moderate-to-severe relapse.

Regarding treatment, the first big question is whether this patient should be hospitalized or not. In this case, it seems appropriate to treat as an outpatient, assuming there is no evidence of fulminant colitis (there isn't... more on that in a later vignette), no signs of sepsis, normal vital signs, and ability to eat. She checks those boxes and is appropriate for outpatient management with close follow-up.

So, what's the best treatment? Let's go through what the guidelines say about the options.

More Mesalamine? Nope. This patient is already on 5-ASAs, and they're not working at the moment. Mesalamine and other 5-ASA products are not appropriate for inducing remission in UC. We need something stronger.

Steroids? Yes. Assuming there are no contraindications, this patient will likely benefit from a limited course of corticosteroids. Research, including controlled studies and meta-analyses, shows that steroids significantly improve outcomes compared to placebo in patients with a UC flare.[41] For more targeted treatment with reduced side effects, budesonide, which has a high rate of first-pass hepatic metabolism, can be effective, particularly in a 9 mg dose. This approach has been validated in clinical trials where budesonide

MMX helped achieve remission by week 8 without increasing adverse events compared to placebo.[42, 43] It's often a good idea to start with budesonide before going to more systemic therapies.

What about thiopurines? Nope. Thiopurines and methotrexate are less effective for inducing remission in moderately to severely active UC. Thiopurines are super slow in onset (takes weeks) and don't reliably induce remission in severe cases. Methotrexate has also shown little benefit for inducing remission, even in higher doses administered intramuscularly.

Anti-TNF Therapies? These therapies can be effective to induce remission in moderate-to-severe UC. Infliximab, adalimumab, and golimumab are all more effective than placebo, but head-to-head trials are lacking. Infliximab shows higher remission rates compared to other anti-TNFs. In network meta-analyses, which use a fancy-dandy statistical technique to estimate how drugs *might* fare if they are pitted head-to-head, there is some evidence that infliximab could have a slight edge compared to adalimumab or golimumab, although the benefit is more of a trend than a statistical certainty.[44, 45] Notably, combo therapy with infliximab and azathioprine is superior to either therapy alone in inducing remission.

Vedolizumab? Yep, this can also work. Earlier, we discussed that vedo is an anti-integrin biologic therapy that is useful for Crohn's. It also has excellent efficacy in UC and can effectively induce remission in moderate-to-severe disease by targeting gut-specific immune responses. This focused action results in a strong safety profile, particularly with fewer infections compared to broader immunosuppressants. In the GEMINI 1 trial, vedolizumab significantly outperformed placebo in achieving clinical remission and mucosal healing by week 6.[46] Further analysis and systematic reviews have reinforced its efficacy, especially in patients previously unresponsive to anti-TNF therapies. Since it is gut selective, some IBD experts prefer using this over more systemic biologics.

Tofacitinib? Yep, this can also work. By the way, there always seems to be yet another option in IBD, which is great for patients, but challenging for non-IBD specialists always working to keep up with the latest therapies and studies ;-). In any event, tofacitinib is an oral Janus kinase (JAK) inhibitor that outperformed placebo in patients with moderate-to-severe UC, particularly those who have failed other therapies.[47] Be aware, however, that infectious complications, especially herpes zoster, were more frequent. For that reason, it is often considered for those who fail less systemic approaches, such as vedolizumab. On the other hand, if there are concurrent autoimmune disease-related skin lesions, like psoriasis, then a more systemic biologic like tofacitinib might be preferred. This is where the art vs science of IBD management comes into play.

Case 1.13: UC Crisis

A 28-year-old woman with a known history of UC presents to the emergency department (ED) with severe symptoms. She reports more than 10 bloody stools per day for the past week, along with severe abdominal pain and cramping. The patient has also had a fever of 102°F, significant fatigue, and a marked decrease in appetite. On exam, she appears pale and tachycardic with a heart rate of 120 beats per minute (bpm) and blood pressure of 90/60 mmHg.

Labs reveal a hemoglobin level of 8.5 g/dL and elevated inflammatory markers, including an ESR of 70 mm/hr and CRP level of 150 mg/L. A stool sample is negative for infectious pathogens. Urgent flexible sigmoidoscopy is performed, showing extensive ulceration, friability, and significant mucosal bleeding extending from the rectum to the descending colon, confirming a severe flare of ulcerative colitis.

Know your guidelines!

How best to manage this patient?

Case 1.13: What do the guidelines say?

Source: ACG 2019 Ulcerative Colitis Guidelines[36]

This patient is in rocky straits with evidence of acute severe ulcerative colitis (ASUC) and requires urgent and close attention. Immediate stool testing is essential to rule out *C. difficile* infection (CDI). Within 72 hours of admission, and preferably within 24 hours, she should undergo a flexible sig to assess the endoscopic severity of inflammation and to obtain biopsies for evaluating CMV colitis, which can be found in up to one third of patients presenting with severe UC, particularly those refractory to corticosteroids.

Continuous assessment for toxic megacolon is crucial during hospitalization. Toxic megacolon is a potentially life-threatening complication characterized by colonic dilation and systemic toxicity.

When evaluating severe colitis with plain abdominal films, look for a thickened colonic wall and loss of haustrations. If you see significant dilation on abdominal imaging, particularly if the transverse colon is >5.5 cm, then that is bad news and needs to be addressed ASAP (**Figure 1.7**).

Keep in mind that ASUC patients should receive deep vein thrombosis prophylaxis (DVT) to prevent venous thromboembolism, as they are at considerably increased risk for a complicated DVT. This should be considered even if the patient is bleeding from colitis, because the more severe the colitis, the higher the risk of a complicated DVT.

Monitoring the response in patients with ASUC should involve tracking stool frequency, rectal bleeding, physical exam (e.g., monitor for peritoneal signs of an acute abdomen), vital signs, and serial CRP measurements. Medications like NSAIDs, opioids, and those with anticholinergic side effects should be avoided due to their potential to exacerbate the condition. Routine use of broad-spectrum antibiotics should be avoided as well unless there is evidence of an intraabdominal infection or sepsis.

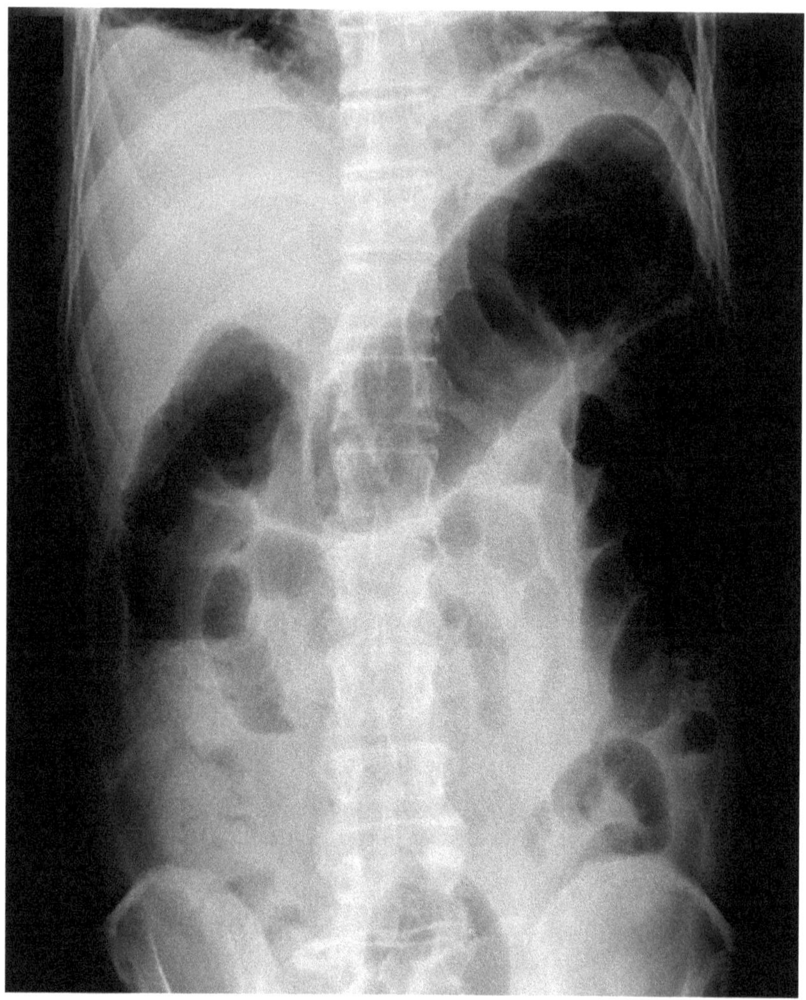

Figure 1.7. *Fulminant colitis with distended colon in ASUC.*
Image from *Gastro Hep Advances.* 2024;3(1):58-59.

In patients who fail to respond adequately to medical therapy by 3-5 days, or in cases of suspected toxicity, surgical consultation is necessary. In general, it's always a good idea to have surgery on board early, and certainly if you see anything like what's shown in Figure 1.7. For medical treatment, methylprednisolone 60 mg/d or hydrocortisone 100 mg 3 or 4 times per day is recommended to induce remission. If the patient does not respond to intravenous corticosteroids within 3-5 days, medical rescue therapy with infliximab or cyclosporine should be initiated.

The choice between infliximab and cyclosporine should depend on provider experience, patient history with immunomodulators or anti-TNF therapy, and serum albumin levels. If the patient achieves remission with infliximab, continue maintenance with the same agent. For those who respond to cyclosporine, maintenance with thiopurines or vedolizumab is suggested. Indications for surgery in ASUC include toxic megacolon, colonic perforation, severe refractory hemorrhage, and poor response to medical therapy. Both infliximab and cyclosporine do not increase postoperative complications of colectomy, so surgery should not be deferred based on these treatments.

More recently, the JAK inhibitors tofacitinib and upadacitinib have been used in ASUC with some success. Their rapid onset and oral delivery contributes to the rationale of their utlility in severe UC when there may be protein leakage from the inflamed bowel that limits success of the protein-based monoclonal antibodies. However, some of the available data are with off-label doses of these therapies and additional ongoing studies will clarify if these treatments may be preferable to cyclosporine or infliximab.

Lastly, total parenteral nutrition for bowel rest is generally not recommended due to the very low quality of evidence supporting its benefit. Regular monitoring for toxic megacolon and careful assessment of treatment response is essential for managing this critical condition.

Case 1.14: Screening Ahead

A 23-year-old man is diagnosed with mild-to-moderate UC extending beyond the rectum to the left colon. Managed successfully on mesalamine, he reports a significant reduction in symptoms with stable disease. His liver tests, including alkaline phosphatase (ALP), are normal, indicating no signs of primary sclerosing cholangitis (PSC). There is no family history of colorectal cancer (CRC). Given the extent and duration of his UC, the patient is advised on the importance of regular colon cancer screening

Know your guidelines!

1. When should you begin CRC screening?

2. How best to screen?

3. What if the ALP had been elevated and there were signs of PSC?

Case 1.14: What do the guidelines say?

Source: ACG 2019 Ulcerative Colitis Guidelines[36]

CRC is a significant concern for patients with UC. Key risk factors include prolonged disease duration, younger age at diagnosis, extensive colonic involvement, higher inflammatory activity and extent of disease, coexisting PSC, and family history of CRC. **Figure 1.8** provides another mnemonic to help memorize these risk factors. Think of a "PEARL" that is slowly growing inside of the colon.

Primary sclerosing cholangitis (PSC)

Extensive colitis

Age at diagnosis (young)

Relative with CRC (family history)

Long disease duration

Figure 1.8. *Risk factors for CRC in UC (spells out PEARL)*

In this case, the patient is young, which raises the risk of subsequent CRC, but there is only mild-to-moderate disease, no PSC, colitis is limited to the left side (i.e., not extensive), and there is no family history of CRC. Thus, the ACG guidelines recommend beginning colonoscopic screening 8 years after the initial diagnosis of UC.

Over the years, the risk of CRC in UC patients has decreased, with estimates showing cumulative risks of 1%, 2%, and 5% after 10, 20, and more than 20 years of disease duration. Regular screening is crucial as CRC in UC typically arises from dysplasia, often presenting as flat lesions rather than polyps, which mandates vigilant monitoring and early detection strategies to improve patient outcomes. Thus, CRC screening in UC must be performed by full colonoscopy, not flex sig, or fecal immunohistochemistry, or other noninvasive forms of stool testing (see *G2G Volume I* for more on CRC screening modalities).

Now, what if this patient had PSC? In that case, you wouldn't want to wait 8 years. You'd need to start right way at diagnosis, followed by yearly checks.

Regular surveillance every 1 to 3 years is recommended based on risk factors and past colonoscopy findings. During exams, the endoscopist should look for raised lesions and abnormal patterns, performing targeted biopsies. If you're using a standard-definition colonoscope, dye spray chromoendoscopy with methylene blue or indigo carmine is recommended to hot-spot dysplasia. With high-definition scopes, white-light endoscopy with narrow-band imaging or dye spray chromoendoscopy can be used. It's essential that a GI pathologist reviews any dysplasia. If dysplasia is completely removed, frequent follow-up colonoscopies are advised, but multifocal or non-resectable dysplasia warrants a proctocolectomy.

Remember, no medical therapy can replace the need for colonoscopic surveillance. Augmented visualization methods, like dye spray chromoendoscopy, can help in ongoing surveillance after detecting dysplasia. Alternative screening methods like fecal DNA testing and CT colonography aren't recommended due to insufficient evidence.

Case 1.15: An Elusive Diagnosis

A 34-year-old woman presents with a 5-year history of IBS-like symptoms, including bloating, abdominal pain, and intermittent diarrhea. Despite trying various therapies such as a low-FODMAP diet, antispasmodics, gut-directed antibiotics, and fiber supplements, her symptoms persist. Recently, her primary care physician noted mild iron deficiency anemia and slightly elevated AST/ALT levels. She is now referred to your GI clinic for further evaluation.

Know your guidelines!

1. What condition are you most worried about?

2. What test should you perform?

Case 1.15: What do the guidelines say?

Source: ACG 2023 Diagnosis and Management of Celiac Disease Guidelines [49]

Given the persistent IBS-like symptoms and additional findings of mild iron deficiency anemia and elevated AST/ALT levels in this patient, it's imperative to test this patient for celiac disease. Studies indicate that approximately 2%-4% of patients with IBS symptoms may have undiagnosed celiac disease. [50] To accurately diagnose celiac disease, an anti-tissue transglutaminase IgA (anti-TTG IgA) antibody test, along with a total IgA measurement, is recommended. The total IgA test is crucial to avoid false negatives, as some individuals may have selective IgA deficiency, which would render the anti-TTG IgA test unreliable.

The presence of iron deficiency anemia and elevated liver enzymes further raises the suspicion of celiac disease. For more on the overlap between IBS and celiac disease, refer to *G2G Volume I* where we cover it in some depth.

Taking a step back, celiac disease is a chronic inflammatory bowel disease that affects approximately 1% of the population worldwide. It's triggered by the ingestion of gluten, a protein found in wheat, barley, and rye, leading to an immune response that damages the small intestinal mucosa. By the way, is gluten found in oats? No, it isn't. But oats are often processed in facilities that also handle wheat, barley, and rye, which can lead to cross-contamination. So, people with celiac need to be careful about eating oats, too, unless they were specifically labeled as being processed in a gluten-free facility.

While we're at it, what other grains do not contain gluten? **Table 1.5** provides a list.

Table 1.5. *Example grains that do not contain gluten.*

Buckwheat
Corn
Millet
Quinoa
Rice (White, brown, wild)
Sorghum

In people with celiac disease, the damage from gluten exposure can impair nutrient absorption, leading to various gastrointestinal and systemic symptoms. Many patients present as if they have IBS, so ACG guidelines recommend routinely screening for celiac disease among patients with IBS symptoms. Also think about testing in people with chronic GI symptoms who have unexplained osteoporosis, infertility, lymphoma, elevated liver tests, and other comorbid complications.

One of your authors once saw a vibrant, 90-year-old woman in his clinic who had lifelong abdominal pain and diarrhea. She was born in France, had been diagnosed with osteoporosis years ago, and lamented never being able to bear children. She was sent to the GI clinic because of iron deficiency anemia. Alas, she had celiac disease, and it's a darned shame she wasn't diagnosed years earlier. It's never too late to think about celiac.

Okay, so how to make the diagnosis of celiac disease? The ACG guidelines focus on testing with the anti-TTG IgA antibody. Those with an elevated TTG IgA should then undergo endoscopic biopsy of the small intestine. On the other hand, if the anti-TTG IgA is negative, you need to also check the total IgA levels to confirm it's not a false negative. If total IgA levels are normal and anti-TTG IgA is negative, then there is a very low chance of there being celiac disease. On the other hand, if the total IgA is low then you cannot

Be sure to check total IgA levels alongside anti-TTG IgA when testing for celiac disease to avoid false negative results from IgA deficiency yet rule out celiac disease. In that case, the guideline recommends testing with an IgG serology, such as the deamidated gliadin peptide (DGP) or anti-TTG IgG antibody.

Now, what if you have a patient with a high pre-test probability of celiac disease, but who has a negative anti-TTG IgA and normal total IgA? Although the negative predictive value is high for this situation it's not 100%. If you suspect celiac disease, particularly if you think the chance is greater than 5% (which isn't all that high, really...), then the guidelines recommend proceeding to endoscopy nonetheless. In this vignette, for example, the patient with IBS symptoms, has not responded to typical therapies, has iron deficiency anemia, and elevated liver tests. This patient should be seriously considered for celiac even if the serology is negative. The ACG guidelines say to still get an upper endoscopy with duodenal biopsies in a case like this.

What about this situation: a patient has already gone on a gluten-free diet even before serologic testing and wants to know if they have celiac disease. What do you do? In this case, the anti-TTG IgA might be falsely negative given the sustained gluten free diet, so you need to try another approach. Rather than ruling in celiac with a serology, you should rule out celiac by checking a human leukocyte antigen (HLA) DQ2/DQ8 haplotype. If negative, you can rule *out* celiac. There is essentially a 100% negative predictive value if this comes back negative. If positive, however you can't really know either way, forcing you to keep moving through the diagnostic algorithm. Start with a 2-week dietary challenge of 3g gluten daily. If the patient can tolerate the diet, then continue for up to 6 additional weeks, and then perform serologic testing at the end of the challenge. If positive, then proceed to endoscopy with biopsy. **Figure 1.9** provides the entire ACG algorithm for diagnosing celiac disease, including additional information about children not mentioned in the text, above.

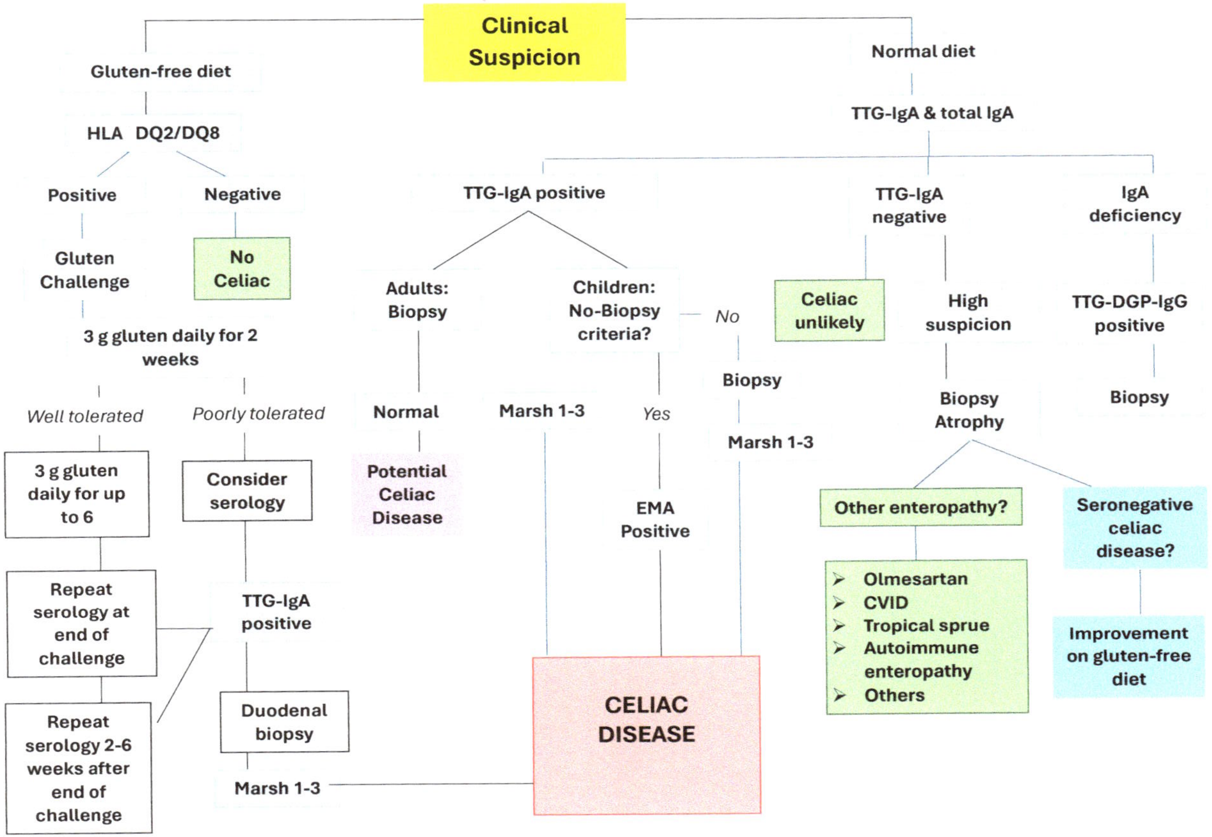

Table 1.9. *Celiac disease diagnostic testing algorithm from ACG guidelines.*[49]

When it comes to endoscopy with biopsy, the key is to perform enough biopsies in the right places. It's crucial to take multiple biopsies of the duodenum due to the patchy nature of histological abnormalities. One study found that submitting 4 or more specimens significantly increased the probability of diagnosing Celiac Disease (1.8% vs 0.7%).[51] However, only 39% of patients had 4 or more biopsies taken. That's pretty weak. I mean, you're already in the duodenum, so why skimp on the biopsies! While you're at it, be sure to take 1-2 biopsies from the duodenal bulb because this can boost the chances of diagnosing celiac. And then, take another 4 or more from the distal duodenum.

The biopsy examines the presence of Marsh lesions, which are classified into four types, demonstrated in **Figure 1.10.**

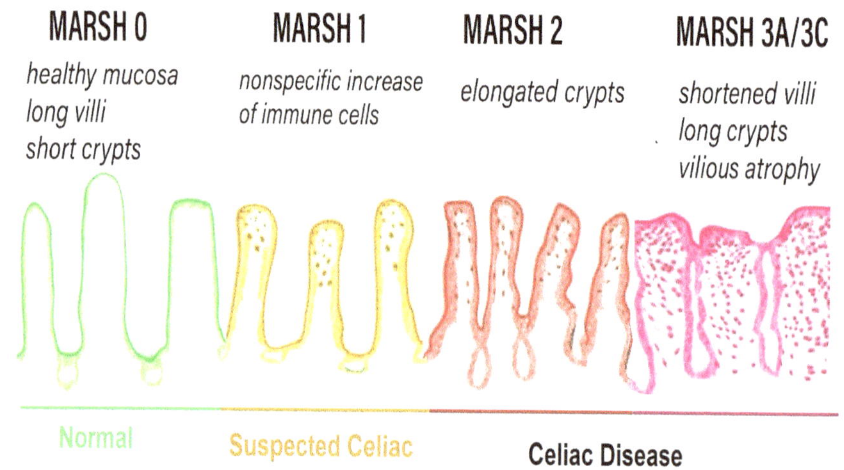

Figure 1.10. *Marsh lesions, ranging from March 0 (normal mucosa) to Marsh 3 (villous atrophy). Increased intraepithelial lymphocytes are found in Marsh 1, along with lymphocyte infiltration with elongated crypts in Marsh 2. Celiac requires March 1-3 lesions to be found on biopsy.*

By the way, does anything else cause villous blunting other than celiac disease? You bet! Think about autoimmune enteropathy, small intestinal bacterial overgrowth (SIBO), graft vs host disease, Zollinger-Ellison syndrome, chronic variable immunodeficiency (CVID), and even Crohn's disease. They can all blunt the villi, too.

The primary treatment for celiac disease is a strict, lifelong gluten-free diet, which typically leads to symptom resolution and mucosal healing. Adherence to the diet is crucial, as even small amounts of gluten can trigger symptoms and mucosal damage. Regular follow-up and dietary counseling are essential to ensure compliance and address any nutritional deficiencies.

Of note, it is not useful to follow serologies after diagnosis, as they are not a reliable indicator of disease status. Although seroconversion to negative serology is possible while on a sustained gluten-free diet, there is no guarantee that will occur. In contrast, sustained presence of anti-TTG IgA does not correlate with symptoms. Thus, serial biopsies are the best way to monitor disease status. The guidelines recommend performing follow-up biopsy 2 years after starting a gluten-free diet.

By identifying and treating celiac disease early, patients can significantly improve their quality of life and avoid long-term complications associated with untreated celiac disease.

Inflammatory Bowel Diseases Quiz

1. Which age group is most commonly affected by the first peak of Crohn's disease onset?

    a) 0-10 years
    b) 15-30 years
    c) 30-45 years
    d) 50-80 years

2. How many individuals in the United States are estimated to have Crohn's disease?

    a) 8,000
    b) 80,000
    c) 800,000
    d) 8 million

3. What enteric infection should be considered due to its overlapping symptoms with Crohn's disease and a propensity for the terminal ileum and cecum?

    a) *Salmonella enterica*
    b) *Campylobacter jejuni*
    c) *Yersinia enterocolitica*
    d) *Shigella dysenteriae*

4. What is a significant limitation of using CRP and ESR levels in diagnosing IBD?

    a) They can both be elevated in IBS
    b) They have long half-lives
    c) Up to 40% of IBD patients with mild inflammation may have normal levels
    d) While ESR can accurately distinguish IBS from Crohn's disease, CRP cannot

5. Which genes are integral to the innate immune response and main-tenance of the intestinal barrier in Crohn's disease?

   a) NOD2, IL-23 receptor, and ATG16L1
   b) BRCA1, BRCA2, and TP53
   c) MTHFR, FTO, and APC
   d) HLA-B27, TNF, and IL-10

6. Which serological marker is more commonly associated with ulcer-ative colitis?

   a) ASCA
   b) ANCA
   c) CRP
   d) ESR

7. Which serological marker is more frequently positive in patients with Crohn's disease?

   a) ASCA
   b) ANCA
   c) ANA
   d) RD

8. Which of the following is not a risk factor for progressive disease burden in Crohn's disease?

   a) Older age at diagnosis
   b) Initial extensvie bowel involvement
   c) Ileal involvement
   d) Perianal disease
   e) Visceral adiposity

9. Above what value does fecal calprotectin after surgery indicate risk of postoperative recurrence?

   a) 50 µg/g
   b) 100 µg/g
   c) 150 µg/g
   d) 200 µg/g
   e) 250 µg/g

10. Which of the following is a <u>not</u> consistently positive risk factor for triggering Crohn's disease flare?

   a) NSAID exposure
   b) *C. difficile* infection
   c) Smoking
   d) Antibiotic exposure
   e) Stressful life experience

11. A 25-year-old woman presents with a 3-month history of intermittent abdominal pain and diarrhea. She has no significant past medical history and does not report recent travel or antibiotic use. A colonoscopy reveals inflammation confined to the terminal ileum, consistent with Crohn's disease. Her laboratory results are unremarkable, except for mildly elevated CRP. Which of the following is the most appropriate initial treatment?

   a) Budesonide
   b) Infliximab
   c) Methotrexate
   d) Azathioprine
   e) Mesalamine

12. A 45-year-old man presents with a 6-month history of severe abdominal pain, frequent diarrhea, and significant weight loss. He reports that his symptoms have progressively worsened, and he now experiences approximately 10 loose bowel movements per day, often with blood. A colonoscopy shows extensive inflammation, deep ulcerations, and stricturing throughout the ileum and ascending colon. His laboratory results reveal elevated CRP and

ESR levels, indicating active inflammation. Which of the following is the most appropriate initial treatment?

a) Budesonide
b) Prednisone
c) Azathioprine
d) Infliximab

13. A 27-year-old woman with a Crohn's disease presents for a follow-up visit. She was initially treated with a course of prednisone which successfully induced remission. However, she has experienced multiple flare-ups requiring courses of budesonide and has been unable to wean off steroids for an extended period. Which of the following is not appropriate next step in her management is:

a) Adalimumab
b) Infliximab
c) Metronidazole
d) 6-Mercaptopurine (6-MP)

14. A 40-year-old man with moderate-to-severe Crohn's presents for evaluation of biologic therapy. He has had an inadequate response to conventional treatments, including corticosteroids and immunomodulators. He is now being considered for infliximab. His medical history is significant for past hepatitis B virus (HBV) infection, which was treated and resolved. Recent screening tests show that he has positive HBsAb and HBcAb, but his HBsAg is negative. Which of the following is the most appropriate course of action?

a) Proceed with infliximab without any additional treatment
b) Start antiviral prophylaxis with entecavir or tenofovir and monitor liver function tests regularly while initiating infliximab
c) Use corticosteroids alone to manage Crohn's disease and avoid biologic therapy
d) Delay infliximab until HBV is treated for 6 months

15. A 25-year-old woman with Crohn's disease is about to start treatment with infliximab. Which of the following vaccines are required prior to starting biologics?

   a) Pneumococcal vaccine
   b) Herpes zoster vaccine (Shingles)
   c) Human papillomavirus (HPV) vaccine
   d) Influenza vaccine
   e) Hepatitis A and B vaccines
   f) All of the above

16. Which of the following best reflects the risk of lymphoma among patients receiving anti-TNF therapy?

   a) 2 per 10,000
   b) 4 per 20,000
   c) 6 per 10,000
   d) 12 per 10,000

17. Which of the following is the mechanism of action for vedolizumab?

   a) Anti-TNF
   b) Anti-a4 Integrin
   c) Anti-IL12/23
   d) JAK inhibitor
   e) Selective adhesion molecule inhibitor

18. Which of the following is the mechanism of action for ustekinumab?

   a) Anti-TNF
   b) Anti-a4 Integrin
   c) Anti-IL12/23
   d) JAK inhibitor
   e) Selective adhesion molecule inhibitor

19. Which of the following is the mechanism of action for golimumab?

    a) Anti-TNF
    b) Anti-a4 Integrin
    c) Anti-IL12/23
    d) JAK inhibitor
    e) Selective adhesion molecule inhibitor

20. Which of the following is the mechanism of action for tofacitinib?

    a) Anti-TNF
    b) Anti-a4 Integrin
    c) Anti-IL12/23
    d) JAK inhibitor
    e) Selective adhesion molecule inhibitor

21. A 31-year-old man with Crohn's disease initially responded well to infliximab 5 mg/kg. However, he is now experiencing a flare-up of symptoms 5 weeks after his last infusion. Endoscopy shows ongoing inflammation, and tests for infections are negative. His lab results show undetectable trough levels of infliximab and no antibodies against the drug. What is the most appropriate next step in his management?

    a) Switch to adalimumab
    b) Increase the dose of infliximab
    c) Add methotrexate
    d) Start prednisone

22. A 29-year-old woman with Crohn's disease, previously well-controlled on infliximab 5 mg/kg, presents with abdominal pain and diarrhea 8 weeks after her last infusion. Stool studies for pathogens and tests for antibodies to infliximab are negative. Laboratory results show detectable infliximab trough levels. What is the most appropriate next step in her management?

    a) Increase the dose of infliximab
    b) Switch to ustekinumab
    c) Add azathioprine
    d) Start budesonide

23. A 34-year-old man with a known history of Crohn's disease presents with mild pain around the anus but no fever or systemic symptoms. An MRI reveals a small perianal abscess less than 5mm in size, without any fistulous tracts. The patient is currently on mesalamine for maintenance therapy. What is the most appropriate next step in managing his condition?

a) Start oral antibiotics and observe
b) Surgical drainage of the abscess
c) Initiate infliximab therapy
d) Monitor the patient closely without immediate intervention

24. A 37-year-old man with Crohn's disease presents with mild discomfort around the anus but no fever or systemic symptoms. An MRI reveals a simple perianal fistula that minimally involves the sphincter muscles. The patient is currently on 6-MP for maintenance therapy. Which of the following is the most appropriate next step in managing his condition?

a) Surgical intervention to repair the fistula
b) Start oral antibiotics
c) Initiate infliximab therapy
d) Start oral prednisone

25. Which of the following is not a risk factor for post-operative recurrence of Crohn's disease:

a) Smoking
b) Use of NSAIDs
c) Limited bowel resection
d) Pre-surgical use of corticosteroids
e) Penetrating or fistulizing disease

26. A 28-year-old woman with UC presents for a routine follow-up. She reports occasional mild rectal bleeding and increased stool frequency, averaging three bowel movements per day. She does not report fever, abdominal pain, or weight loss. A recent colonoscopy showed mild inflammation limited to the rectum and sigmoid colon, with a Mayo score of 1. What is the most appropriate treatment for this patient?

a) Start corticosteroids

b) Initiate infliximab therapy

c) Prescribe mesalamine

d) Begin azathioprine

27. Which of the following is not a risk factor for poor UC prognosis?

   a) Age >40 at diagnosis

   b) Mayo score of 3 or greater

   c) Elevated CRP

   d) Low serum albumin

   e) Extensive colitis

28. A 45-year-old man with a UC presents to the ED with severe abdominal pain, distension, and bloody diarrhea. He has experienced a rapid decline in his condition over the past 48 hours, including high fever, tachycardia, and hypotension. Physical exam reveals a tender, distended abdomen with reduced bowel sounds. Labs show elevated white blood cell count, anemia, and severe electrolyte imbalances. An abdominal X-ray reveals colonic dilation to 8 cm. What is the most appropriate next step in managing his condition?

   a) Start high-dose corticosteroids and monitor closely

   b) Initiate infliximab therapy

   c) Administer broad-spectrum antibiotics

   d) Emergency surgery

29. Which of the following is not a risk factor for CRC in UC?

   a) Family history of CRC

   b) Long disease duration

   c) Extensive colitis

   d) Older age at diagnosis

   e) Co-morbid primary sclerosing cholangiopathy

30. In the absence of PSC, when should colonoscopic CRC screening begin after the initial diagnosis of UC?

   a) Screen immediately
   b) In 1 year
   c) In 2 years
   d) In 4 years
   e) In 8 years

31. A patient with celiac disease adheres strictly to a gluten-free diet but continues to have symptoms. What is the most likely reason for persistent symptoms?

   a) Refractory celiac disease
   b) Small intestinal bacterial overgrowth
   c) Lactose intolerance
   d) Non-compliance with the gluten-free diet
   e) Microscopic colitis

32. Which nutritional deficiencies are commonly associated with celiac disease?

   a) Vitamin B12, iron, and vitamin D
   b) Vitamin C, potassium, and magnesium
   c) Calcium, sodium, and phosphorus
   d) Vitamin K, folate, and iodine

33. A patient with celiac disease who has been on a strict gluten-free diet presents with a pruritic, blistering rash on the elbows and knees. What is the most likely diagnosis?

   a) Atopic dermatitis
   b) Dermatitis herpetiformis
   c) Psoriasis
   d) Contact dermatitis

34. Which of the following grains does not include gluten?

a) Maize
b) Wheat
c) Barley
d) Rye

35. A 40-year-old woman presents with chronic diarrhea, bloating, and weight loss. There is no iron deficiency anemia or family history of celiac disease. Testing shows negative anti-TTG IgA. However, her total serum IgA level is found to be low. What is the most appropriate next step in diagnosing celiac disease in this patient?

a) Assume it is not celiac disease and look for other causes
b) Test for anti-endomysial antibodies
c) Check deamidated gliadin peptide antibodies
d) Perform a small bowel biopsy immediately

36. A 35-year-old man presents with chronic diarrhea, bloating, iron deficiency anemia, and elevated liver enzymes. He has not responded to typical therapies for IBS. Celiac disease is highly suspected. Serological testing shows negative anti-TTG IgA and normal total IgA levels. What is the most appropriate next step in diagnosing celiac disease in this patient?

a) Reassure the patient and manage symptoms as IBS
b) Perform genetic testing for HLA-DQ2/DQ8
c) Proceed with an upper endoscopy and duodenal biopsies
d) Check deamidated gliadin peptide antibodies

37. A 30-year-old woman presents with a history of chronic gastrointestinal symptoms and has been on a self-initiated gluten-free diet for the past 6 months. She wants to know if she has celiac disease. Her initial serological testing for anti TTG-IgA is negative with a normal total IgA level. What is the most appropriate next step in diagnosing celiac disease in this patient?

a) Reassure the patient and maintain the gluten-free diet

b) Perform genetic testing for HLA-DQ2/DQ8

c) Start a 2-week dietary challenge of 3 g gluten daily and repeat serology

d) Proceed directly to endoscopy with biopsy

38. A 28-year-old man was recently diagnosed with celiac disease and has started a strict gluten-free diet. He has been compliant with the diet and reports an improvement in his symptoms. You are planning his follow-up care. What is the most appropriate follow-up strategy for this patient?

a) Monitor serologies every 3 months

b) Perform a repeat small bowel biopsy in 2 years

c) Conduct genetic testing for HLA-DQ2/DQ8 annually

d) Schedule routine endoscopies every 6 months

Answers to Inflammatory Bowel Diseases Quiz

1.	B	20.	D
2.	C	21.	B
3.	C	22.	B
4.	C	23.	D
5.	A	24.	B
6.	B	25.	C
7.	A	26.	C
8.	A	27.	A
9.	B	28.	D
10.	D	29.	D
11.	A	30.	E
12.	B	31.	D
13.	C	32.	A
14.	A	33.	B
15.	F	34.	A
16.	C	35.	C
17.	B	36.	C
18.	C	37.	B
19.	A	38.	B

CHAPTER TWO

UNINVITED GUESTS

Navigating the Landscape of GI Infections

Consider yourself as a donut for a moment. When you thread your finger through a donut's center, you're traveling through the core without ever actually being within the donut's substance. Organisms with an intestinal tract function similarly. Their digestive tube is an inversion of their body, running straight through from front to back. It's a continuous channel, and while the body envelops this channel, nothing within the channel is technically "inside" the organism in the same way that threading your finger through a donut doesn't place it inside the pastry. Or, if donuts aren't your thing, think of those slippery "Water Wiggler" toys that elude your grasp by folding inward on themselves; that's also a tube-within-a-tube design just like the intestines inside your body. It should come as no surprise that our tubes get infected pretty easily. Afterall, they are *directly* exposed to the outside world. Were it not for stomach acid, we'd directly instill billions of bacteria into our gut every time we ate a sausage. As an important aside, that's one reason to be a little careful about long-term use of proton pump inhibitors (PPIs), a topic we cover in *G2G Volume I*.

So, with all of that in mind, let's talk about GI infections. There are all sorts of "uninvited guests" that invade our bowels, and this chapter will cover some of them. We'll start with the #1 gut pathogen, prevalent in so many people worldwide, and that's *H. pylori*. Then, we'll discuss *C. difficile*, a prevalent and challenging infection to manage. The chapter will wrap up with a discussion about acute diarrhea infections in travelers. So, hold on to your microbiome and get ready to talk buggers.

Case 2.1: Persistent Dyspepsia and *H. pylori* Infection

A 43-year-old man has been experiencing dyspepsia for 8 months, characterized by postprandial burning in the epigastrium, but without retrosternal burning or regurgitation. He reports no nausea, vomiting, unintended weight loss, or rectal bleeding. Labs do not show anemia, abnormal liver tests, or other biochemical abnormalities. A stool antigen test for *H. pylori* (HP) returns positive. The patient has never before been tested or treated for HP, has no recent antibiotic exposures, and is not allergic to penicillin.

Know your guidelines!

1. How should this patient be treated?

2. What are the chances of eradicating the HP with 1 round of therapy?

3. What are the chances that eradicating HP will help manage the dyspepsia?

Case 2.1: What do the guidelines say?

Source: ACG 2024 *H. pylori* Guidelines[52]

Before we dive into the management of this case, let's take a moment to appreciate the fascinating backstory of HP's discovery—a tale of scientific curiosity, personal sacrifice, and eventual Nobel Prize recognition. Barry Marshall, alongside Robin Warren, embarked on a journey that would forever alter our understanding of gastric diseases. In a bold move that blurred the lines between experimenter and experiment, Marshall ingested HP himself, developing gastritis as a result. This daring act provided compelling evidence of HP's role in causing peptic ulcers and challenged the prevailing medical dogma that ulcers were primarily caused by stress or spicy food. We both remember learning in medical school that ulcers were a sign of neuroticism, but that turned out to be wrong. Very wrong. Instead, the groundbreaking work of Marshall and Warren revealed that most ulcers were caused by an infection—a truly remarkable insight at the time—and illuminated a path for treating and preventing a range of gastrointestinal disorders, earning them the Nobel Prize in Physiology or Medicine in 2005.

As for the epidemiology of HP, it's been a companion of humanity for over 100,000 years. This bug is quite the globetrotter, with subpopulations tracing our own migrations across continents. HP is the most common chronic bacterial infection worldwide, affecting more than 40% of us globally. That's just wildly common. The good news is that its prevalence has been on a slow decline—from over 58% a few decades ago to around 43% more recently—although it still clings on stubbornly, particularly in places where resources are scarce. Lifeforms have a way of persisting at all costs.

In North America, about 30%-40% of the population harbors HP, with its presence more common among certain groups.[50] Unfortunately, it is an infection of disparities, seen more frequently in non-White races and ethnicities, those living in crowded conditions or with poorer sanitation, and among immigrants from areas where the bacteria are widespread. The infection usually takes up residence in childhood, setting the stage for various gastric troubles down the line, from dyspepsia to ulcers, and increasing the risk for gastric cancer.

Anyway, let's talk about this patient. We already discussed the dyspepsia guidelines in depth in Volume I of the G2G series, so check back there for details. We'll keep it concise here. In short, the ACG recommends an HP "test and treat" strategy as the first-line approach for cases of uninvestigated dyspepsia where no alarm features, such as unintended weight loss or rectal bleeding, are present and the patient is under 60 years of age.

Our patient here fits neatly into this recommendation. With eight months of dyspepsia symptoms but no alarm features, testing for HP is warranted. The subsequent positive stool antigen test triggers the "treat" portion of the "test and treat" guideline. This approach is based on the understanding that, for many patients, eradicating HP can improve dyspepsia symptoms. Meta-analysis reveals that test and treat for HP lowers the symptoms of dyspepsia by 25%, on average, compared to using placebo ($P= 0.0005$).[54]

HP eradication lowers symptoms of dyspepsia by 25% on average

The guideline's straightforward directive—"test and treat," not "test and then think more about whether or not you want to treat"—simplifies the decision-making process, ensuring prompt and effective care. So, whenever you test for HP, it should be with the expectation that you plan to treat if the test comes back positive. Don't test and then get all wishy washy if the test comes back positive.

Beyond dyspepsia, what are the other indications to test for and treat HP? The list is long and shown in **Table 2.1**. Naturally, any patient with a peptic ulcer should be tested for HP and offered treatment if positive. Same with marginal zone B-cell lymphoma. Patients with unexplained iron deficiency anemia should also be tested for HP, along with idiopathic thrombocytopenic purpura (ITP), which in some cases is linked to HP infection.

Table 2.1. *Indications for HP test and treat.*

Groups to test and treat for *H. pylori* infection[1]
Peptic ulcer disease: prior history or active disease
Marginal zone B-cell lymphoma, MALT type
Uninvestigated dyspepsia in patients who are under the age of 60 years
In high-risk populations for gastric cancer, test and treat at age 45-50 years
Functional dyspepsia
Adult household members of individuals who have a positive non-serological test for *H. pylori*
Patients taking long-term NSAIDs or starting long-term treatment with low-dose aspirin
Patients with unexplained iron deficiency anemia
Patients with idiopathic (autoimmune) thrombocytopenic purpura
Primary and secondary prevention of gastric adenocarcinoma
Current or history of gastric premalignant conditions[2]
Current or history of early gastric cancer resection
Current or prior history of gastric adenocarcinoma
Patients with gastric adenomas or hyperplastic polyps[3]
Persons with a first degree relative with gastric cancer[4]
Individuals at increased risk for gastric cancer including certain non-White racial/ethnic groups, immigrants from high gastric cancer incidence regions/countries, hereditary cancer syndromes associated with an increased risk for gastric cancer[4]
Patients with autoimmune gastritis
[1] In the absence of contraindications, *H. pylori* treatment should be offered to all patients with active *H. pylori* infection, as indicated by a positive non-serological test. Serological testing is not recommended in low prevalence populations in the absence of a high pre-test probability (e.g., peptic ulcer). [2] GPMC include atrophic gastritis, intestinal metaplasia, and dysplasia. [3] Patients with adenomas and hyperplastic polyps often have associated GPMC. [4] A decision to test and treat should follow shared decision-making between the patient and provider.

Okay, so this patient tested positive, which means you've got to offer treatment. There are many available treatment regimens for HP, so how do you decide which one to use? The decision depends, in part, on whether the patient is treatment-naïve, whether they have allergies to certain antibiotics (e.g., penicillin), and their previous exposure to macrolides. But to keep things simple, the ACG guidelines recommend bismuth quadruple therapy (BQT) as first line for all treatment-naïve patients.

BQT Therapy. This regimen includes a bismuth salt, a nitroimidazole (typically metronidazole, but could use tinidazole), tetracycline (not doxycycline), and a PPI. Although some previous regimens used a histamine-2 receptor antagonist (H_2RA) instead of a PPI, the ACG guidelines do not recommend use of H_2RAs in treating HP.

One large study of 585 patients demonstrated an 87% eradication rate of HP using BQT over 14 days.[55] Reducing the treatment duration to 10 days or substituting doxycycline for tetracycline notably decreased its effectiveness. So, keep that in mind. Don't prescribe 10-day courses of anti-HP therapy, and don't substitute doxycycline for tetracycline. This contrasts with the PPI-clarithromycin triple therapy, whose eradication rates have declined due to rising clarithromycin resistance, now seen in approximately 32% of U.S. cases.[56] Despite the fall in triple therapy eradication rates, that regimen still is the most commonly prescribed first-line HP therapy. The ACG guidelines reommend we use BQT instead, since it works better.

BQT is favored over the triple therapy, especially given its efficacy in the face of clarithromycin resistance—a significant hurdle for the latter, as evidenced by both U.S. and European studies and meta-analyses.[57] The absence of amoxicillin in BQT also makes it suitable for patients with penicillin allergy. Despite its advantages, including bypassing the need for antimicrobial sensitivity testing, BQT's drawbacks include a large number of pills, potential side effects, and challenges related to the cost and availability of tetracycline.

Rifabutin-Based Triple Therapy. There are other regimens that the ACG guidelines suggest are reasonable as first line therapies. For example, rifabutin triple therapy, combining a PPI, rifabutin, and amoxicillin, has now expanded from a choice for those previously treated for HP to also include treatment-naïve patients. Despite limited comparison with other first-line treatments, this regimen stands out for its low resistance rates and the lack of clarithromycin, side-stepping concerns over macrolide resistance without needing pre-treatment sensitivity checks. The potential for myelo-toxicity, a known risk with rifabutin, appears mitigated at the doses used in the current anti-HP regimen. Further research comparing rifabutin triple therapy directly to other treatments like BQT could illuminate its place in HP management strategies.

Potassium-Competitive Acid Blocker (PCAB) Regimens. Vonoprazan, a PPI alternative that works through potassium-competitive acid blockade, offers a fresh approach to treating HP, especially in dual therapy with amoxicillin. Its action on gastric acid secretion outperforms PPIs, maintaining a higher intragastric pH that boosts antibiotic efficacy against HP.[58] The FDA has approved vonoprazan in 2 formulations for HP treatment, highlighting its ease of use—no meal timing constraints—and effectiveness even in clarithromycin-resistant strains.

Key studies underscore its merits: In one trial by Chey and colleagues, vonoprazan-amoxicillin matched the eradication rates of a standard triple therapy and showed superior results against clarithromycin-resistant HP.[59] Research from China further supports its use, demonstrating non-inferiority to more complex regimens.[60] The simplicity of vonoprazam-based dual therpy, combined with not needing to perform antibiotic resistance testing, make it a compelling option for first-line treatment, although the guidelines currently list it as "conditional," whehreas BQT is supported by "strong" evidence.

The conversation around gastric acid suppression in HP treatment also touches on genetic factors like CYP2C19 metabolism rates, affecting PPI effectiveness. However, with vonoprazan's entry, there is no need to navigate these genetic considerations, simplifying treatment choices and potentially reshaping strategies for HP eradication.

Table 2.2. provides a list of other anti-HP treatment regimens along with the level of recommendation per the ACG guidelines.

Regimen	Drugs (doses)	Dosing frequency	FDA Approval	Recommendation
Bismuth quadruple	PPI (standard dose)	b.i.d.	No	STRONG (moderate quality of evidence)
	Bismuth subcitrate (120 - 300 mg) or sub-salicylate (300 mg)	q.i.d.		
	Tetracycline (500 mg)	q.i.d.		
	Metronidazole (500 mg)	tid or q.i.d..		
Rifabutin triple (Talicia™)	Omeprazole (10 mg)	4 capsules t.i.d.	Yes	CONDITIONAL (low quality of evidence)
	Amoxicillin (250 mg)			
	Rifabutin (12.5 mg)			
PCAB dual (Voquezna DualPak™)	Vonoprazan (20 mg)	b.i.d.	Yes	CONDITIONAL (moderate quality of evidence)
	Amoxicillin (1000 mg)	t.i.d.		
PCAB triple (Voquezna TriplePak™)	Vonoprazan (20 mg)	b.i.d.	Yes	CONDITIONAL (moderate quality of evidence)
	Clarithromycin (500 mg)			
	Amoxicillin (1,000 mg)			

Table 2.2. *Recommended regimens for treatment-naïve patients with HP infection.* b.i.d., twice daily; FDA, US Food and Drug Administration; PCAB, potassium channel acid blocker; PPI, proton pump inhibitor; q.i.d., 4-times daily; t.i.d., 3-times daily.

The ACG guidelines emphasize that, in the U.S. and other parts of the world, HP is increasingly resistant to clarithromycin and levofloxacin, leading to a drop in treatment success rates to 70% or less with these antibiotics. That's not good. Clarithromycin resistance, in particular, means standard treatments often fail to eradicate HP. Given these resistance issues and the World Health Organization's call for careful use of these antibiotics, it's advised to steer clear of regimens based on clarithromycin or levofloxacin, especially without confirming the strain's susceptibility. While these drugs can still be an option for certain patients, the serious side effects tied to fluoroquinolones, like levofloxacin (especially tendon rupture), emphasize the need for cautious selection and consideration of alternatives like amoxicillin, tetracycline, and rifabutin, which have much lower resistance rates.

The ACG guidelines also suggest to only use clarithromycin for HP if the strain is known to be sensitive, and to consider alternatives if susceptibility testing isn't available. This is a major change over previous guidelines and reflects a more judicious approach to using clarithromycin in this era of increasing resistance. In patients without prior macrolide use and where clarithromycin must be used, opt for a 14-day regimen with a PCAB rather than a PPI, as studies show PCAB-based therapies provide better eradication rates, especially against clarithromycin-resistant strains. However, the real challenge is when clarithromycin sensitivity is unknown; here, PCAB-clarithromycin triple therapy could be preferable to its PPI counterpart.

In short, for patients newly facing HP and lacking antibiotic susceptibility data, the go-to is 14-day optimized BQT. Rifabutin triple therapy or 14-day PCAB dual therapy are viable choices for those without a penicillin allergy. For patients with no prior macrolide exposure or penicillin allergy, a 14-day PCAB-clarithromycin triple therapy is favored over the PPI-clarithromycin equivalent.

Case 2.2: Persistent Dyspepsia After *H. pylori* treatment

The patient in the last vignette receives BQT therapy for 14 days. The epigastric pain moderately improves during the treatment period, but then returns within a week of completing therapy.

Know your guidelines!

1. Why did the symptoms improve and then worsen again?

2. Should you confirm HP cure? If so, how?

Case 2.2: What do the guidelines say?

Source: ACG 2024 *H. pylori* guidelines[52]

This patient with uncomplicated dyspepsia underwent appropriate testing and treatment for HP. While eradicating HP can decrease dyspepsia symptoms by roughly 25%, it's not uncommon for bothersome symptoms to persist that can impact quality of life. This could be due to HP not being the primary cause or to failure to eradicate. The symptom improvement during BQT is likely due to the high-dose PPI component, suggesting acid sensitivity. The return of symptoms post-treatment suggests that PPI therapy might be beneficial long-term. However, it's crucial to verify whether HP was eradicated, mandating further testing.

After treating HP, it's essential to confirm whether the therapy worked. You should use either a urea breath test, fecal antigen test, or gastric biopsy—at least four weeks after finishing treatment. Since acid blockers like PPIs and possibly PCABs can mess with test results, leading to false negatives, patients should take a break from them for at least two weeks before testing. And don't forget, antibiotics and bismuth need a four-week pause too. Serology tests won't help here—they can wave the HP flag long after the organism is gone.

Sometimes, especially for serious cases like a big ulcer or gastric MALT lymphoma (i.e., not in this case), you might end up scoping the stomach anyway after treatment. If so, you can grab biopsies to check the HP status on the spot (always get at least 2 biopsies from the antrum, and 2 from the mid-body, greater curve, for maximum yield). Just remember, the sensitivity drops if the patient recently took PPIs, PCABs, bismuth, or antibiotics.

Skipping the post-treatment confirmation of cure is a no-go. We need to make sure the HP is gone so we don't leave patients open to more trouble down the road. Plus, patient-reported symptoms don't always match up with whether the treatment eradicated the HP. So, test after treatment, no matter what.

This isn't just about the patient in front of you—there are bigger issues at play. The ACG guidelines emphasize that routine eradication testing helps track how well treatments are working over time. If success rates dip, then it's time to rethink our strategy, maybe check for drug resistance, or switch up the treatment game plan. It's great that post-treatment testing has shot up from only 25% to 60-80% in recent years, but let's keep pushing for 100%.

Case 2.3: Persistent *H. pylori* Despite Treatment

Continuing with the same patient as before, you check a stool antigen test with the patient off PPI therapy and discover that it's still positive. The patient also continues to report persistent meal-related epigastric pain.

Know your guidelines!

How should you proceed?

Case 2.3: What do the guidelines say?

Source: ACG 2024 *H. pylori* guidelines[52]

As HP eradication rates have been on the decline, it's important to have a plan for when initial treatments don't cut it. Luckily, the ACG guidelines provide clear next steps for handling HP when first-line therapies don't achieve the desired outcome.

If the bug hangs around after the first round of treatment, then our next step, according to the guidelines, is to call in the big guns second line therapies. Which set of big guns depends on what treatment the patient already received. **Figure 2.1** provides an algorithm for how to proceed with "salvage therapy" when first line treatment fails.

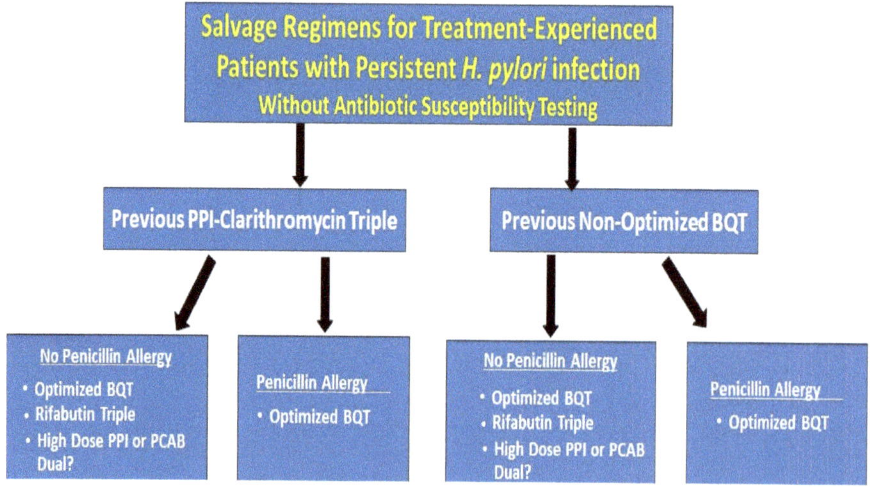

Figure 2.1. *Recommended regimens "salvage therapy" after initial treatment failure. Note that all of these should last for 14 days.* [52]

In this case, the patient received optimized BQT, so that is a nonstarter for second line therapy. However, it's important to know that many people still do not receive optimized BQT first line, but instead are prescribed either another form of triple therapy or receive a course of "non-optimized" BQT, where the treatment is too short and/or the doses are too low. In those cases, the ACG guidelines recommend "optimized" BQT therapy, which is a beefed-up version of the regular regimen, lasting 14 days with bismuth, metronidazole, tetracycline (remember...not doxycycline), and a PPI. See **Table 2.3** for the dosing details of this optimized BQT along with other available second-line regimens.

Despite hurdles like the common side effects of tetracycline, the guidelines still back optimized BQT as the go-to for second attempts at beating HP. The guideline authors are wary of using clarithromycin or levofloxacin in the absence of targeted susceptibility testing, especially with resistance on the rise and black box warnings about levofloxacin's risks. Sticking to the rule of thumb, if someone's had macrolides or fluoroquinolones before, do not use them again for HP. Yet, it turns out many patients get the same treatment twice, leading to repeated treatment failures and pointing to a need for better practices and patient education in managing HP.

In short, if HP persists after the first treatment round and the patient has not yet tried optimized BQT, then that's the suggested 14-day plan. But if optimized BQT's off the table, then rifabutin triple therapy for 14 days is the next line of defense. Before reaching for clarithromycin or levofloxacin, the guidelines recommend susceptibility testing to see if the bacteria are sensitive to those meds, a topic we'll discuss in the next vignette. If tests show sensitivity to clarithromycin and it hasn't been used before, a well-dosed triple therapy with a PPI or PCAB is worth a shot for another 14 days. Levofloxacin can also be considered if it's a new option for the patient and the bacteria are susceptible, keeping in mind the associated safety warnings regarding tendon and nerve damage. When it comes to high-dose dual therapy, though, the guidelines emphasize that we don't yet have any evidence to recommend dual therapy in North America.

Regimen	Drugs (doses)	Dosing frequency	AST Required?	Recommendation
Optimized-Bismuth quadruple	PPI (standard dose)	b.i.d.	No	CONDITIONAL (very low quality of evidence)
	Bismuth subcitrate (120 - 300 mg) or sub-salicylate (300 mg)	q.i.d.		
	Tetracycline (500 mg)	q.i.d.		
	Metronidazole (500 mg)	tid or q.i.d..		
Rifabutin triple	PPI (standard to double dose)	b.i.d.	No	CONDITIONAL (low quality of evidence)
	Amoxicillin(1,000 mg)	b.i.d. or t.i.d.		
	Rifabutin(50-300 mg)	q.d., b.i.d., or Talicia™ which contains 50 mg t.i.d.)		
Levofloxacin triple	PPI (standard dose)	b.i.d.	Yes	CONDITIONAL (low quality of evidence)
	Levofloxacin (500 mg)	q.d.		
	Amoxicillin (1,000 mg) or metronidazole (500 mg)	b.i.d.		
PCAB triple (Voquezna TriplelPak™)	Vonoprazan (20 mg)	b.i.d.	Yes	No recommendation (evidence gap)
	Clarithromycin (500 mg)			
	Amoxicillin (1000 mg)			
High dose dual therapy	Vonoprazam (20 mg) or PPI (double dose)	b.i.d. or t.i.d.	No	No recommendation (evidence gap)
	Amoxicillin(1,000 mg)	t.i.d.		

Table 2.3. *Recommended regimens "salvage therapy" after initial treatment failure.* [52]

Note that all of these should last for 14 days.

AST, antibiotic susceptibility testing; b.i.d., twice daily; PCAB, potassium channel acid blocker; PPI, proton pump inhibitor; q.i.d., 4-times daily; t.i.d., 3-times daily.

Case 2.4: Susceptibility Testing for *H. pylori*

Let's keep running with the previous vignette. Now, the patient received a second-round treatment with rifabutin-based triple therapy for 14 days. The dyspepsia persists, and *H. pylori* antigen testing, off PPIs, reveals persistent positivity.

Know your guidelines!

How should you proceed?

Case 2.4: What do the guidelines say?

Source: ACG 2024 *H. pylori* guidelines[52]

This is a situation that comes up more and more. It's important to know how to respond to multiple failed attempts at HP eradication, and once again, the ACG guidelines have us covered.

When things get tough, it's important to move away from the one-size-fits-all treatment approach and consider susceptibility testing and tailored therapy. Testing comes in two flavors: traditional cultures and more cutting-edge molecular techniques. While cultures are more classic, they're tricky to perform and not very common due to their fussiness and unpredictability. HP is a rather fastidious organism that can be hard to grow.

To collect and transport gastric biopsies for HP culture, ensure the biopsies are taken from both the antrum and body of the stomach. Do your best to use sterile techniques to avoid contamination. Place the biopsies immediately into a transport medium suitable for HP to maintain viability. The sample should be kept at room temperature and sent to the laboratory as quickly as possible, ideally within a few hours of collection, to enhance the chances of successful culture growth.

In contrast to traditional culture and sensitivity, molecular methods, like polymerase chain reaction (PCR), shine a spotlight on specific gene mutations linked to drug resistance, offering a quicker, often more accessible way to tailor treatments. Next-generation sequencing (NGS) is yet another approach that can survey multiple resistance markers at once, boosting the chances of picking the right antibiotic from the get-go.

Deciding among culture, PCR, or NGS for HP susceptibility testing hinges on effectiveness, cost, and practicality, with molecular methods showing promise for spotting specific resistance mutations. The high DNA yield from NGS might edge out traditional cultures in reliability. However, the real-world choice depends on what's accessible and affordable locally.* Despite numerous trials exploring the efficacy of ta ilored antibiotic t eatments, di verse methodologies across studies make direct comparisons tough, highlighting a gap in understanding best practices for integrating susceptibility testing into treatment plans. In short, the ACG guidelines recommend employing antibiotic susceptibility testing, although it's best performed locally, whenever the choice of therapy remains unclear after taking into consideration previous treatments for HP, past antibiotic exposure more generally, and whether there is a documented history of penicillin allergy. **Figure 2.2** summarizes the recommended approach to interpreting antibiotic susceptibility testing for HP.

*NOTE The term "real world" comes up a lot in research studies, but it's a funny term, right? Like, as opposed to some alternative or fake world or "the Upside Down" for you *Stranger Things* fans out there. Anyway...

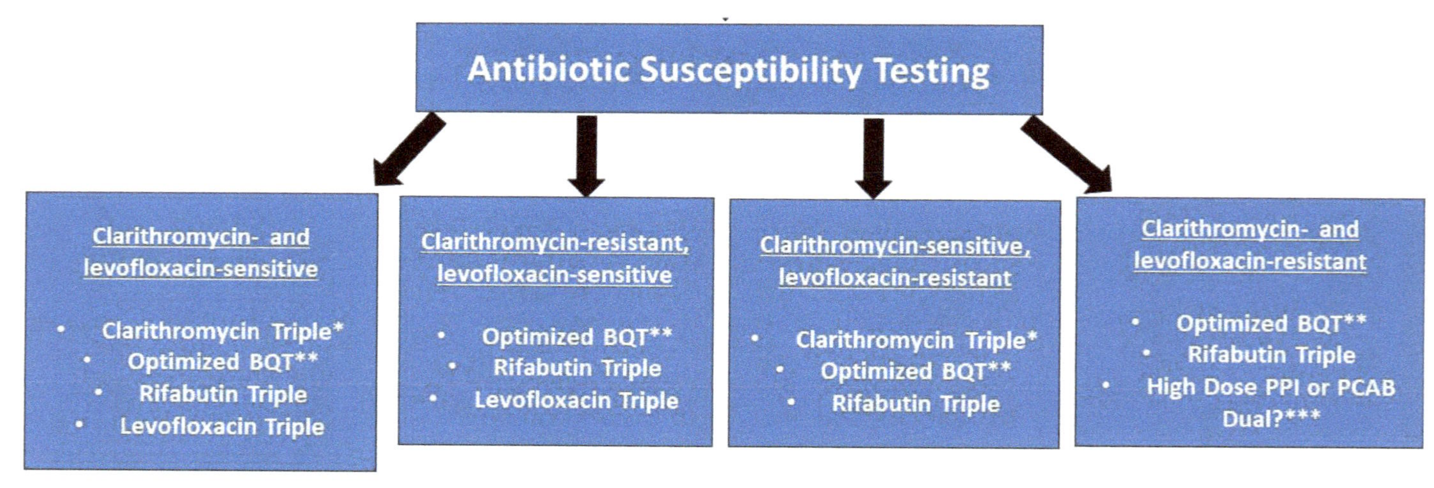

Figure 2.2. *Salvage regimens for treatment-experienced patients with persistent H pylori infection without antibiotic susceptibility testing. Approach to using antibiotic susceptibility testing for HP salvage therapy selection.*

Case 2.5: *C. difficile* in a Nursing Home

An 82-year-old female nursing home resident with advanced dementia recently started experiencing upper abdominal pain related to meals. She has not vomited, has no evidence of rectal bleeding, and no diarrhea or incontinence of stool. The primary care physician at the nursing home ordered a variety of tests, including an abdominal ultrasound that was unremarkable, a complete blood count that was normal, and stool studies that returned a positive test for *C. difficle*. You are now being consulted to manage this finding.

Know your guidelines!

How should you proceed?

Case 2.5: What do the guidelines say?

Source: ACG 2021 *Clostridioides difficile* guidelines[61]

Okay, raise your hand if you've ever had a patient with *C. difficile*. Are you raising your hand? No? Okay, fair enough. But if you're a gastroenterologist, or really any kind of doctor, then you probably see too much *C. difficile*. Way too much. I mean, even *psychiatrists* see too much *C. difficile*!

If you take care of patients, then this vignette, and the next several to follow, are for you. Let's learn how to manage this common infection, starting with distinguishing true infection from mere colonization.

Previously, guidelines suggested testing for *C. difficile* when someone is experiencing 5-6 loose stools in a day, but now the bar is set at only 3. The ACG guidelines emphasize testing in cases of new, unexplained diarrhea but also acknowledge that in certain settings, like upon admission to high-risk transplant or oncology units, testing can help with lowering the overall burden of infections. Remember, finding *C. difficile* doesn't always mean there's an active infection; many carry the bug without symptoms.

That's the main point of this vignette. This patient may come from a high prevalence setting, but she has no diarrhea at all. There's an old clinical saw that if stool doesn't take the shape of the container in which it's contained, then it probably shouldn't be tested for *C. difficile*. In this case, testing was inappropriate, because there are zero symptoms of true infection. Meal related dyspepsia is not a classic symptom of *C. difficile,* and lack of diarrhea is pretty much an exclusion. This is probably just colonization, so treatment is not indicated.

That said, there are occasional situations where it's reasonable to test for *C. difficile* in the absence of diarrhea. For example, if someone has new onset, otherwise unexplained ileus or Ogilvie's in a high-risk environment, like an intensive care unit (ICU) or bone marrow transplant unit, then the guidelines suggest it might be warranted to test. But in general, unless someone has 3 or more unformed stools over 24 hours, the pre-test probability of active *C. difficile* infection—in contrast to colonization—is low, and testing should be minimized. In this case, testing for *C. difficile* was not appropriate, so treatment should not be initiated.

Case 2.6: Diagnosing *C. difficile* in a Hospitalized Patient

A 69-year-old man, hospitalized for recurrent pneumonia and on IV antibiotics, now reports 5 episodes of unformed, non-bloody stools daily. His vital signs reveal a maximum temperature of 100.4°C without evidence of hypotension. His bowel sounds are reduced but present, and abdominal imaging has not revealed ileus. Laboratory findings include a white blood cell count of 12,000 cells/μL, serum creatinine at 1.2 mg/dL (slightly elevated from his baseline of 1.0 mg/dL), and normal electrolyte levels. You are now consulted by the primary medical team "to perform a colonoscopy."

Know your guidelines!

1. Is a colonoscopy warranted at this time?

2. You are concerned about *C. difficile* infection. What stool study should you order?

Case 2.6: What do the guidelines say?

Source: ACG 2021 *C. difficile* guidelines[61]

In contrast to the previous case, this patient is clearly at risk for *C. difficile* infection (CDI) and is passing unformed stool. Your Spidey sense for CDI should be high, and formal testing is appropriate.

So, what do the ACG guidelines recommend for diagnosing *C. difficile*? The key points are shown in **Figure 2.3**.

When a patient shows signs of CDI, start with a broad net—a highly sensitive test like the glutamate dehydrogenase (GDH) assay or nucleic acid amplification test (NAAT)—to catch any hint of the bug. This first step quickly weeds out false alarms. Both the GDH and NAAT tests are 96% sensitive for catching CDI with a 100% negative predictive value. So, if either of these tests is negative, you can rest assured there's no *C. difficile*, assuming the sample was properly collected.

On the other hand, if either of these first-line tests return positive, then you can't yet know for sure there is CDI because the positive predictive value ranges from around 34% to 46%.[63] In other words. There's less than a 50% chance of actual CDI in the presence of a positive GDH or NAAT test. Moreover, the GDH test does not distinguish toxigenic from non-toxigenic strains of *C. difficile,* so even if the bug is present, it's not necessarily toxigenic. That's why we need another step to close the loop.

In the presence of a positive GDH or NAAT, the next step is the toxin EIA—a much more specific test that confirms if the bug is not just present, but also causing trouble by producing toxins. The EIA specifically looks for toxins A and B produced by *C. difficile*. It's 99% specific, but far less sensitive which is okay since the initial tests take care of sensitivity. This 2-tiered approach helps strike a balance, ensuring we treat the real cases and not the harmless carriers.

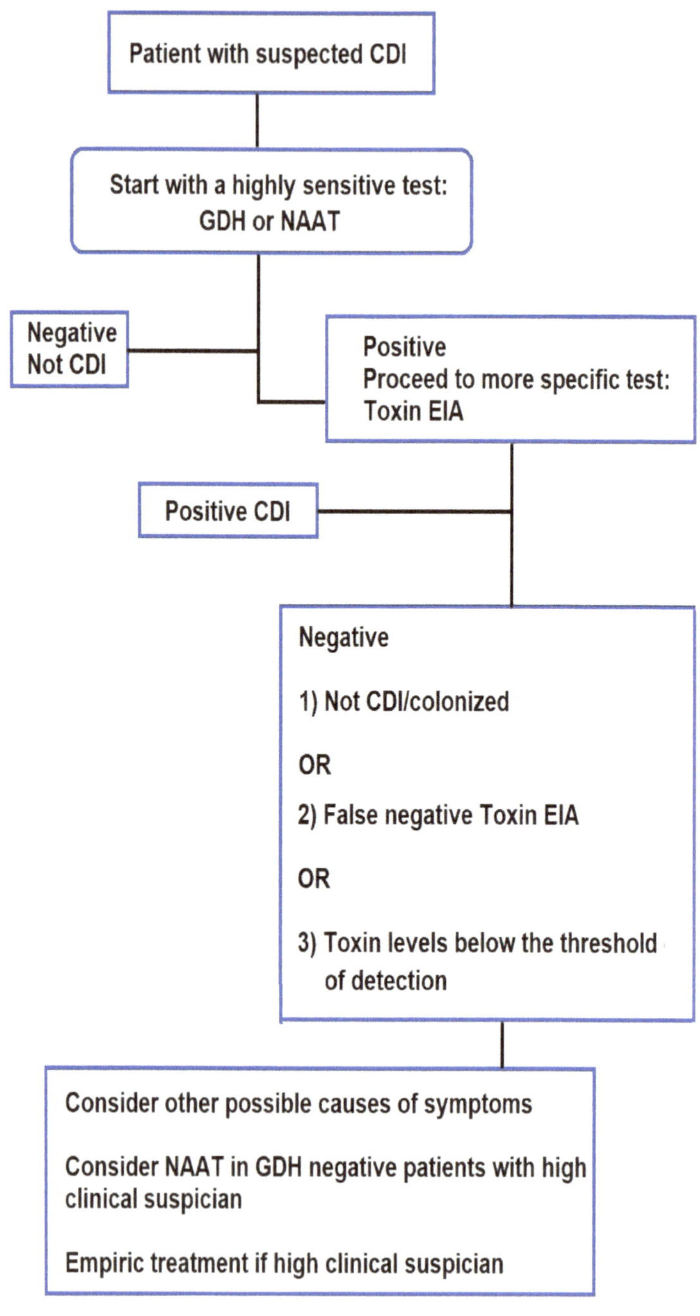

Figure 2.3. *ACG Guidelines Algorithm for C. difficile Testing*

We face a dilemma when the highly sensitive GDH or NAAT tests are positive, but the specific toxin EIA is negative. It could mean a patient is just a carrier, or they have CDI with low toxin levels that the test couldn't pick up. Because tests aren't infallible, it is vital to employ clinical expertise to make the call. If you strongly suspect CDI based on the overall picture, risk factors, and clinical symptoms, then you might opt to treat regardless of a negative toxin EIA result, assuming the initial screening test is positive.

What about the request for a colonoscopy? Should we scope right away? No, not really. CDI can be noninvasively diagnosed using the testing algorithm we just discussed and does not mandate invasive examination. If you are on the fence about whether CDI is the cause of diarrhea (e.g., positive GDH or NAAT but negative EIA), then colonoscopy or a flex sig might be warranted to confirm your suspicion. In that case, if you do the colonoscopy, then you will look for the classic pseudomembranous colitis of CDI, shown in **Figure 2.4.** If you don't recognize that image, then I'm afraid we need to take away your GI license if you have one. ;-)

Figure 2.4. *Pseudomembranous colitis of CDI.*

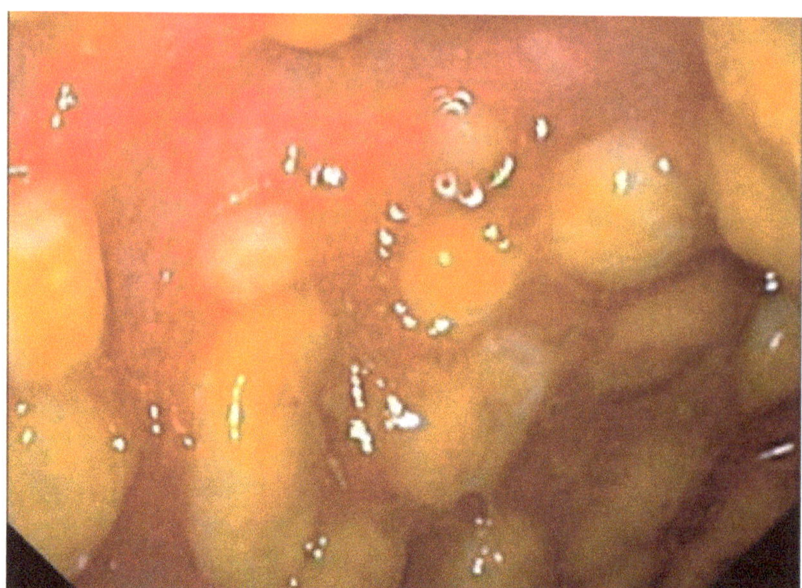

Reprinted from The Lancet, 371. Kuipers and Surawicz. Clostridium difficile infection, 1486-88, ©2008 with permission from Elsevier.

Case 2.7: Treatment of CDI #1

Let's go back to the last case. Take a look at the details again, including the vital signs and lab values. Okay, now, let's assume this patient tests positive for CDI with both a positive GDH and EIA test, indicating active infection. Got it? Okay, then take a look at the questions, below.

Know your guidelines!

1. How do you rate the severity of this case of CDI?

2. How will you treat this patient?

Case 2.7: What do the guidelines say?

Source: ACG 2021 *C. difficile* guidelines[61]

Determining the right treatment path for CDI hinges on assessing the disease's severity. The ACG guidelines underscore that the approach to treatment should be tailored to each case's specifics. Let's review the CDI classification scheme, which will guide us in making informed decisions about this patient's care.

Over the last decade and beyond, experts have been crafting all sorts of clinical prediction rules to forecast the CDI outcomes and optimize treatment. While these rules draw from a mix of clinical signs and lab markers—like age, ICU stays, and white blood cell counts—they aren't perfect. The simpler, the better seems to be the consensus. Both the Infectious Disease Society of America (IDSA) and ACG guidelines indicate CDI is serious if the white blood cell count blows past 15,000 cells/L or if the serum creatinine ex-ceeds 1.5 mg/dL.[64] Later guidelines added more signs of trouble, like shock or ileus. But the proof's in the pudding—or rather, in large studies. One such study used data from the Veteran's Affairs (VA) and found that while these criteria are great at ruling out risk, they're less accurate at pinpointing who's truly at high risk.[65] Until we design something better, the IDSA's guide remains the tool of choice, mainly for its simplicity and practicality. **Table 2.4** summa-rizes this CDI classification scheme.

CDI Severity Category	Supportive Clinical Data
Non-severe infection	WBC ≤15,000 cells/mL and Serum creatinine <1.5 mg/dL
Severe infection	WBC >15,000 cells/mL or Serum Creatinine >1.5 mg/dL
Fulminant infection	Hypotension or shock, ileus, or megacolon

Table 2.4. *IDSA criteria for determining CDI severity.* WBC, white blood cell.

In the current case, the patent has a WBC of 12,000 cells/mL and a serum creatinine of 1.2 mg/dL. There is no evidence of hypotension or shock, no signs of ileus, and no mention of megacolon on abdominal imaging. He has a low-grade fever but otherwise appears to be clinically stable. Thus, applying the IDSA criteria, he can be classified as having non-severe CDI.

So, how best to manage non-severe disease? Once upon a time, the ACG recommended oral metronidazole for mild CDI, but vancomycin was the go-to for the severe cases. Now, the script has flipped. The latest ACG guidelines tip the scales towards vancomycin or fidaxomicin even for non-severe CDI, relegating metronidazole to a backup role, primarily due to accessibility concerns.

Vancomycin is a top contender for treating CDI. It's more effective than metronidazole, with studies showing superior outcomes in both clinical cure and reducing recurrence rates. As a first-line therapy, vancomycin is often preferred due to its potent bactericidal action and the fact that it remains in the gut, where it can directly target the infection without systemic absorption. Given its broad efficacy, vancomycin is particularly recommended for patients with comorbidities, those who are hospitalized, and immunocompromised individuals. However, cost and availability can be limiting factors for some patients. In the ACG guidelines, vancomycin is recommended as a primary treatment option for non-severe CDI due to its enhanced efficacy.

Fidaxomicin, though much pricier, stands shoulder to shoulder with vancomycin on effectiveness while featuring lower recurrence rates. The real benefit is that it's a directed therapy for *C. difficile*, which means it doesn't knock out other commensals like *Bacteroidetes* and *Firmicutes* species which act, in part, to check and balance *C. difficile* by maintaining a diverse microbiome. In contrast, less specific therapies, including vancomycin, are great for *C. difficile*, but also kill other organisms, affecting the overall balance of the microbiome and increasing risk of recurrence should *C. difficile* persist. Various studies have weighed in, from RCTs to cost-effectiveness analyses, suggesting that fidaxomicin's has an important place in therapy.[66] That said, it's darned expensive.

Metronidazole's role for non-severe CDI is debated. The data are conflicting, with some studies showing it on par with vancomycin and others tipping in favor of vancomycin or fidaxomicin. For the younger, healthier outpatients watching their wallets, metronidazole might still do the trick. The ACG guidelines still say it's okay to use metronidazole as first line, but are generally more excited about vancomycin or fidaxomicin due to enhanced clinical efficacy. Because there is increasing resistance to metronidazole, it also should not be used in patients with serious comorbidities, IBD, immunocompromised individuals, and those are are hospitalized. Only non-severe, outpatient, otherwise healthy pateints are eligible for metronidazole. Bottom line: most experts do not recommend metronidazole as first line if other, more effective therapies are accessible, but it's still an option for certain patients.

Rifaximin's foray into CDI treatment as a follow-up to standard therapy showed promise in cutting back on recurrences, but the jury's still out without bigger trials to seal its fate. The ACG guidelines also cite concerns about high resistance rates and thus do not currently recommend this agent for routine first-line therapy. Similarly, **nitazoxanide** has been tried although it too currently has minimal and low quality date supporting its use.

Antimotility agents like **loperamide** used to be a complete no-go, with fears of bottling up the toxins leading to severe complications. However, recent insights suggest that once CDI treatment is underway, they might be safe to take the edge off diarrhea and urgency.

Bile acid binders, meanwhile, sit on the sidelines. They might have some theoretical perks, but without concrete evidence and potential drug interactions with vancomycin, they're not ready for prime time.

In short, it's most reasonable to treat this patient with either vancomycin or fidaxomicin (the latter being more targeted with less recurrence, thus ideal except for its very high price).

Case 2.8: Treatment of CDI #2

A 72-year-old woman with a history of chronic obstructive pulmonary disease presents to the ED with a 3-day history of frequent, watery diarrhea, and abdominal cramping. She recently completed a course of antibiotics for a respiratory infection. On examination, she appears dehydrated with mild tachycardia and abdominal palpation reveals diffuse tenderness. Her labs show a white blood cell count of 18,000 cells/μL and a serum creatinine of 2.0 mg/dL, up from her baseline of 0.9 mg/dL. A stool sample tests positive for *C. difficile*. Given the marked leukocytosis and renal function deterioration, she is admitted for further management.

Know your guidelines!

1. How do you rate the severity of this case of CDI?

2. How will you treat this patient?

Case 2.8: What do the guidelines say?

Source: ACG 2021 *C. difficile* guidelines[61]

This case is more severe than the previous one. Here using the ISDA criteria, the patient meets the definition of severe CDI, as evidenced by having both an elevated leukocyte count and high serum creatinine. She is not overtly hypotensive or obviously septic, but the presence of tachycardia is concerning that the illness is becoming more advanced. This patient needs timely and effective therapy.

For the tough cases of CDI, vancomycin has long been the go-to, and as we saw in the last case, fidaxomicin has now joined the ranks. A comprehensive network meta-analysis suggests that vancomycin is the superior choice for initial cure.[67] Meanwhile, fidaxomicin demonstrates efficacy in reducing recurrences, with cost-effectiveness analyses suggesting a potential balance in value between the two drugs, despite fidaxomicin's higher upfront costs.[68]

Let's talk dosing—turns out more isn't always better. A head-to-head trial of the standard 125 mg against a pumped-up 500 mg of vancomycin showed they're basically in a tie.[69] And even in the most severe cases of CDI, cranking up the vancomycin didn't provide incremental benefits. Therefore, standard dosing remains the recommendation unless clinical circumstances suggest an alternative cause of symptoms.

Even for severe CDI, there is no advantage of high-dose vancomycin vs standard dosing

Metronidazole for severe CDI? That ship has sailed. It's been outrun by vancomycin in the race for effectiveness. Delayed initiation of vancomycin in favor of metronidazole has also been associated with adverse outcomes such as extended hospitalization, increased incidence of acute kidney injury, and lower cure rates. So, vancomycin is favored from the outset for severe CDI, with studies indicating a notable reduction in 30-day all-cause mortality compared to metronidazole.

In short, vancomycin and fidaxomicin are both acceptable first-line treatments for severe CDI, although the ACG guidelines indicate that vancomycin receives a "strong recommendation" while fidaxomicin is given a "conditional recommendation." Guess you'll have to go with your gut on this one!

Case 2.9: Treatment of CDI #3

A 65-year-old man with a history of rheumatoid arthritis, currently on immunosuppressive therapy, presents to the with a 2-day history of profuse watery diarrhea, severe abdominal pain, and marked distension. He reports at least 10 episodes of diarrhea per day and has not been able to keep down any fluids. His past medical history is notable for a recent hospitalization for pneumonia, during which he received a course of broad-spectrum antibiotics.

On exam, he is febrile with a temperature of 102°F, tachycardic with a heart rate of 112 bmp, hypotensive with a blood pressure of 90/50 mmHg, and tachypneic with a respiratory rate of 26 breaths per minute. His abdomen is markedly distended, with diffuse tenderness to palpation, guarding, and absent bowel sounds. Initial laboratory tests reveal a white blood cell (WBC) count of 23,000 cells/μL, a serum lactate of 4.5 mmol/L, and acute renal failure with a creatinine level of 2.8 mg/dL, up from a baseline of 1.0 mg/dL.

A CT scan of the abdomen shows thickening of the colon consistent with colitis and significant colonic distension without perforation. A stool sample returns positive for *C. difficile* toxin. You are called to provide input to the primary medical team who is admitting the patient. They really want you to scope the patient.

Know your guidelines!

1. How do you rate the severity of this case of CDI?

2. How will you treat this patient?

3. Who else needs to be consulted ASAP, and why?

Case 2.9: What do the guidelines say?

Source: ACG 2021 *C. difficile* guidelines[61]

Things are getting serious here. This patient meets criteria not just for severe CDI, but for fulminant CDI. The white count and creatinine are significantly elevated, blood pressure is dropping, and the colon is distended and at risk for catastrophic perforation. This patient is extremely sick, mandating urgent, multidisciplinary care.

Should you scope the patient now? That doesn't seem like a great idea. This colon is already teetering on the edge, so the last thing you should do is insert a scope and perforate. For some reason, we've both been asked by ICU teams, on various occasions over the years, to urgently scope patients like this with fulminant colitis. Don't take the bait. Sure, you might see pseudomembranes and confirm the diagnosis visually, but you might also perforate the bowel at the same time. What's the point of a diagnostic colonoscopy in this case? There's virtually zero point.

Instead, it's vital to adopt a team approach. Early on, get critical care specialists and infectious disease experts on board, and don't hesitate to involve the surgeons. Aggressive fluid resuscitation is key, especially keeping an eye on the kidneys and the urine output. Serial imaging helps to gauge the severity of colitis and to check for any complications like toxic megacolon or perforation.

With really severe CDI, you might ramp up the vancomycin to a 500 mg dose every six hours, though this isn't backed by hard evidence, just informed guesses and consensus-based recommen-dation. However, considering the high stakes of fulminant CDI, this aggressive approach is deemed appropriate initially. If there's clinical improvement within the first 72 hours, the dosage can be reduced. If there's no improvement, the care team should consider alternative strategies. You might even add on intravenous metroni-dazole, especially if there is ileus. Throw everything you've got at it.

There are limited data to support the use of fidaxomicin in fulminant CDI, as its efficacy in this specific patient group has not been well-studied. Other treatments, like intravenous immunoglobulin and colonic lavage with polyethylene glycol, have been explored, but their roles remain unconfirmed, and they are not routinely recommended. The guidelines also suggest that for those with ileus, using vancomycin enemas every 6 hours might also help. The ultimate treatment decisions should be made on a case-by-case basis, weighing the clinical judgment against the available evidence.

What about the role of FMT? FMT has emerged as a promising treatment for severe and fulminant CDI that doesn't respond to standard therapies. While individual FMT treatments cure up to 91% of cases,[70, 71] multiple FMTs, often done in sequence, may be necessary for lasting cures in more severe cases. Sequential FMT protocols have been developed, showing high success rates for severe and fulminant CDI when combined with oral vancomycin. Most of the FMT data is based on colonoscopic instillation, so in this case there is some risk inserting a scope given the risk of perforation. While a diagnostic colonos-copy is not indicated, if you were forced to do therapeutic colonoscopy for purposes of FMT, then use CO_2, avoid looping, and be super careful!

FMT not only improves cure rates but also appears to reduce the need for colectomy, lowers the incidence of CDI-related sepsis, and may enhance survival in critically ill patients. For example, at one center, the introduction of FMT led to a decline in CDI-related colectomies to zero.[72] That's just amazing, isn't it?

For patients who improve enough to be discharged but still have pseudomembranes, oral vancomycin or fidaxomicin continues at home, followed by an outpatient FMT.

Clinical improvement after FMT is monitored by stool consistency, frequency, the absence of pseudomembranes, and normalized inflammatory markers like white blood cell count and CRP levels. While FMT is an important consideration after 48–72 hours of intensive medical therapy, surgery remains a crucial intervention, especially in cases with complications such as toxic megacolon, ischemia, or perforation. Nonetheless, given FMT's less invasive nature and fewer postoperative risks, it is a preferred early option for severe and fulminant CDI.

Case 2.10: Recurrent CDI

A 59-year-old woman with a history of hypertension and type 2 diabetes presents with a 4-day history of watery diarrhea, averaging 6 to 7 unformed stools per day. She reports a recent hospitalization 3 weeks prior, where she was diagnosed with non-severe CDI and completed a 10-day course of oral vancomycin with resolution of symptoms.

She does not report any abdominal pain, fever, nausea, or vomiting. There is no blood or mucus in the stool. She mentions feeling fatigued and having unintentional weight loss of about 5 lbs since her last hospital discharge. She confirms she has been adherent to her diabetes medication and has not been on any new antibiotics since the last episode of CDI.

On physical exam, she is afebrile with stable vital signs. Her abdominal exam is notable for mild diffuse tenderness without rebound or guarding, and there are no palpable masses. Bowel sounds are present and normoactive.

Lab tests show a WBC count of 12,000/uL, which is elevated compared to her baseline. A repeat stool test for CDI is positive. Her renal function is within normal limits, and there are no electrolyte imbalances. Her HbA1c indicates good glycemic control.

Know your guidelines!

How will you treat this patient?

Case 2.10: What do the guidelines say?

Source: ACG 2021 *C. difficile* guidelines[61]

FMT has significantly changed the game for patients with recurrent *Clostridioides difficile* infection (rCDI), offering a high success rate for those who have battled through multiple rounds of traditional antibiotics without lasting relief. This method works by not only addressing the immediate infection but also reducing the likelihood of recurrence—a major win in the battle against rCDI.

The evidence for FMT's effectiveness comes from a robust body of research, including randomized controlled trials that compare FMT not only against sham placebo, but also versus active treatments like vancomycin and fidaxomicin.[73, 74] What stands out in these studies is FMT's ability to achieve a cure with significantly lower rates of recurrence, positioning it as a highly effective treatment option, especially for rCDI.

When deciding how best to administer FMT for rCDI, there are two main options: oral capsules vs direct instillation via colonoscopy or enema. Another option for the upper GI tract route involves direct instillation via enteroscopy. However, there is an increased risk of aspiration of the contents that you need to consider. At any rate, each approach offers pros and cons.

Opting for capsules presents a convenient and non-invasive route. The ease of swallowing a capsule (assuming no esophgeal obstruction or dysphagia), without the need to visit a hospital or endure a procedure, is attractive for many patients. It avoids the discomfort and preparation associated with more invasive methods, aligning with the preference of patients favoring simplicity and minimal intervention. The effectiveness of capsule delivered FMT, supported by research, stands on par with direct instillation. That's pretty compelling in favor of capsules.

> FMT delivered via oral capsule vs direct colonic instillation are equally efficacious for rCDI

But not everyone is excited to ingest capsules filled with donor fecal material, a psychological hurdle that can be challenging to overcome. It's important that we do not stigmatize this therapy or make patient feel as if it's experimental, or unusual, or disgusting. When done correctly, FMT is a safe, effective, and evidence-based treatment for CDI.

Dosing precision can also prove elusive, potentially requiring multiple administrations to achieve the desired therapeutic effect. Moreover, the logistics of storing and handling these biologically active capsules demand careful attention to maintain the microbial viability essential for treatment success.

As for direct instillation, this approach offers its own set of advantages. This method ensures that the microbiota make direct contact with the colonic lining, a factor that might enhance the effectiveness of the treatment. The ability to visually inspect the colon during the procedure adds a layer of diagnostic value, allowing clinicians to identify and address other potential issues.

Yet, direct instillation is not without its drawbacks. The invasiveness of the procedure, requiring either colonoscopy or enema, may deter some patients. The associated discomfort, the need for bowel prep, and the risks of any invasive procedure contrast with the simplicity of capsule therapy. Additionally, the logistical and resource implications of organizing these procedures, including the availability of skilled practitioners and the costs involved, can be significant.

In navigating the choice between capsules and direct instillation for FMT, patients and clinicians must engage in thoughtful dialogue and shared decision making. Considering the patient's medical history, treatment preferences, and the logistical aspects of each option, a tailored approach that prioritizes patient comfort and treatment efficacy emerges as the guiding principle.

On the safety front, FMT has a reassuring profile. While minor, transient symptoms like abdominal discomfort or bloating are common, serious adverse events are rare, underscoring FMT's safety in a clinical setting. This safety, combined with its efficacy, makes FMT a compelling option for those facing recurrent infections.

Despite the overall success, FMT isn't foolproof, and there's a small chance of FMT failure, where the initial treatment doesn't lead to a lasting cure. In these instances, repeating the FMT or considering alternative delivery methods can often lead to success. This iterative approach underscores the importance of persistence and adaptability in managing rCDI.

Overall, the ACG guidelines emphasize that FMT is a significant advancement in treating rCDI, offering hope and a high rate of success for those who have endured recurrent infections. With its strong safety and efficacy profile, FMT is a valuable tool in the fight against this challenging condition, marking a significant shift towards more effective and durable treatment strategies.

Finally, in managing rCDI in those who aren't eligible for FMT, have relapsed post-FMT, or frequently need antibiotics, long-term suppressive oral vancomycin can effectively stave off further episodes. Additionally, oral vancomycin prophylaxis during subsequent systemic antibiotic treatments offers a strategy to mitigate recurrence risks in patients with a prior CDI history, particularly those at heightened risk of recurrence. This approach balances the prevention of rCDI against the potential for promoting antibiotic resistance and disrupting gut microbiota

Case 2.11: CDI on PPIs

A 53-year-old woman with a history of significant gastroesophageal reflux disease (GERD), well-controlled on PPIs, recently completed a course of antibiotics for an upper respiratory infection. Following antibiotic treatment, she developed symptoms consistent with CDI, including frequent, unformed stools without blood, and abdominal cramping. Stool testing confirmed the presence of *C. difficile* toxins, leading to a diagnosis of non-severe CDI. She was started on oral vancomycin, with symptomatic improvement noted within several days.

However, her primary care physician is now concerned about the ongoing use of PPIs in the context of CDI. The provider is aware of potential associations between PPI use and increased risk of CDI and seeks your input on whether the PPI therapy should be discontinued, adjusted, or continued as is, given her significant GERD symptoms.

Know your guidelines!

Should you stop the PPI?

Case 2.11: What do the guidelines say?

Source: ACG 2021 *C. difficile* guidelines[61]

There's evidence suggesting that gastric acid suppression from PPIs may increase the risk of both primary and recurrent CDI. This is supported by a systematic review of over 7,000 patients which found those on acid suppression therapy had a higher rate of CDI compared to those not using these medications.[75] The FDA has also recognized the potential link between PPI use and CDI, highlighting the difficulty in completely ruling out this association due to factors like age, other illnesses, and antibiotic use which also elevate CDI risk.

It's important to approach these data with caution, considering patients on PPIs often have other risk factors for CDI. The theory is that PPIs might change the gut microbiome or diminish the protective role of gastric acid, facilitating infection from ingested pathogens. However, a major trial involving over 17,000 participants found only a marginal increase in enteric infections among PPI users over three years, with a small difference in CDI cases that wasn't statistically significant.[76] So yes, there is a signal there. But is it large enough to stop PPI use in a patient like this?

The ACG guidelines say that while there's a slight potential risk of CDI with PPI use, the effect is minor compared to other well-established risk factors. Stopping PPI therapy might pose more risk by leaving acid-related GI conditions untreated. Therefore, it's advised to evaluate the need of PPI therapy in CDI patients carefully. If PPIs are deemed necessary for valid medical reasons, their benefits significantly outweigh the slight risk of CDI. In this case, it's probably okay to continue the PPI given the significant benefits in quality of life and GERD symptom abatement from the therapy.

Case 2.12: IBD and CDI

A 32-year-old woman with a known history of UC presents to your office with a 1-week history of increased bloody diarrhea, abdominal pain, and a recent weight loss of 5 pounds. She reports 6 to 8 bowel movements daily, significantly higher than her usual baseline of 1 to 2 semi-formed stools per day. She reports no recent travel, dietary changes, or antibiotic use. Her UC had been well-controlled on infliximab until this recent flare.

On examination, she is afebrile with stable vital signs. Abdominal examination reveals mild left-sided tenderness without rebound or guarding. Laboratory workup shows a mild increase in CRP and ESR, and stool studies are notable for both an elevated fecal calprotectin level and positivity for *C. difficile*.

Given the worsening of her symptoms and the positive *C. difficile* test, a colonoscopy is performed to assess the extent of her UC flare and rule out CDI-related pseudomembranous colitis. The colonoscopy reveals continuous colonic inflammation consistent with UC, extending from the rectum to the splenic flexure. Notably, there are no pseudomembranes seen.

Know your guidelines!

1. Should you treat the *C. difficile*? Or is this just colonization?

2. Should you stop the infliximab?

3. What is the role of FMT in IBD-related CDI?

Case 2.12: What do the guidelines say?

Source: ACG 2021 *C. difficile* guidelines[61]

As we discussed in Chapter 1, it's always important to check for CDI whenever a patient with IBD has a flare. The ACG guidelines emphasize this strongly, and point to research from Manitoba (where Charles Bernstein and colleagues have been doing amazing IBD research for years) highlighting that individuals with IBD exhibit a nearly 5-fold increased likelihood of developing CDI compared to those without IBD, with similar risks observed between UC and Crohn's disease.[77] Factors such as steroid use, biologic therapies, frequent healthcare interactions, and a shorter IBD history elevate the CDI risk.

IBD patients facing CDI often require escalated IBD treatment and incur higher healthcare utilization rates. While the overall mortality risk from CDI may be lower in the ambulatory IBD population, IBD patients hospitalized with CDI face significantly increased mortality risks—especially those with UC. This heightened risk emphasizes the importance of timely CDI management in hospitalized patients.

> IBD patients hospitalized with CDI face significantly increased mortality compared to those without CDI

Interestingly, IBD patients with CDI seldom present with pseudomembranes on endoscopy, complicating the diagnosis and severity assessment of CDI. In the current case, the patient has no pseudomembranes despite testing positive for *C. difficile*, raising the question about whether this is mere colonization vs CDI. But since you've now read this book, you'll know in the future to not be fooled. It's vital to assume this is CDI and treat accordingly.

> IBD patients with CDI often do not have pseudomembranes

As for the best treatment, the guidelines recommend vancomycin 125mg by mouth 4 times daily for a minimum of 14 days, not the more common course of 10 days. Fidaxomicin has too little data

> Treat CDI in IBD for 14 days, not 10 days

for the guideline to recommend at this time for managing CDI in IBD, so stick with vancomycin.

Finally, if an IBD patient develops CDI while on immunosuppressants (as in this case), the guidelines emphasize that the IBD treatment should not be held during anti-CDI therapy. Keep treating the UC while simultaneously managing the CDI.

What about the role of FMT in IBD-related CDI? Could FMT help, or possibly worsen IBD symptoms. This has been an area of great interest in the IBD community, particularly since rCDI is rather common in these patients. Just as with non-IBD patients with rCDI, those with IBD and multiple bouts of CDI can indeed benefit from FMT, with high success rates.

Nonetheless, despite its efficacy in clearing CDI, a subset of IBD patients (7%–25%) experience worse symptoms post-FMT, sometimes requiring increased immunosuppressive treatment or surgical intervention.[78] These observations emphasize the need for careful patient selection and monitoring. However, a notable prospective study of IBD patients with rCDI highlighted a 91% success rate in CDI eradication with FMT, with two-thirds of participants seeing an improvement in their IBD symptoms.[79] This suggests FMT's safety and effectiveness in the IBD population mirrors that in non-IBD patients, making it a viable option for managing recurrent CDI in IBD sufferers.

Case 2.13: Traveler with Diarrhea

A 34-year-old woman presents to the ED complaining of 5-6 loose, watery, non-bloody stools per day for the past 72 hours. She recently returned from a 2 week vacation in Surat, India, where she recalls eating spicy street food on several occasions. She also mentions that she has been feeling generally unwell, with a low-grade fever peaking at 100°F and experiencing bouts of nausea without vomiting and central abdominal discomfort. Physical examination reveals mild abdominal cramping without rebound or guarding, but she is tachycardic with a heart rate of 102 bpm. She reports no recent antibiotic use, and her past medical history is unremarkable. She is adequately hydrated but expresses concern over her persistent symptoms and the impact on her ability to care for her young children at home.

Know your guidelines!

1. What diagnoses are most likely?

2. What diagnostic tests should you perform?

3. How will you treat this patient?

Case 2.13: What do the guidelines say?

Source: ACG 2016 Acute Diarrheal Infections Guidelines[80]

This patient has acute diarrhea after traveling to a region with endemic diarrheal pathogens. Infectious diarrhea is likely. To help determine the most likely pathogen, it's important to first figure out if this is more of a small bowel, malabsorptive-type diarrhea, or large-bowel, colitis-type diarrhea. How can you tell them apart? **Table 2.5** provides some tips.

Table 2.5. *Clinical features to help distinguish small bowel vs large bowel source of acute diarrheal illness. These are just rules of thumb and not definitive, but they can help form a clinical impression even before diagnostic testing.*

Clinical Feature	Small Bowel Origin	Large Bowel Origin
Volume of stool	Larger volume	Smaller volume
Blood in stool	Non-bloody	Bloody
Location of pain	Central	Lower
Relationship of pain to stool passage	Variable	Improves with stool passage
Presence of fever	Variable	More likely
Proctitis symptoms (frequency, urgency, incontinence)	Less Likely	More likely

Small bowel diarrhea typically presents as high volume and watery, with discomfort often centered in the abdomen. Unlike colitis, which can cause bloody, smaller-volume diarrhea and may be accompanied by a higher degree of fecal urgency or even incontinence, small bowel diarrhea generally lacks these symptoms (but they can still occur). In cases of colitis, diarrhea may be more frequent, potentially due to proctitis, and abdominal pain, usually in the lower abdomen, might temporarily subside post-defecation. Although fever can accompany both conditions, its presence might be more indicative of colonic involvement due to an invasive organism.

In the scenario described, the patient experiences watery, voluminous, non-bloody diarrhea with central abdominal discomfort and only a low-grade fever, without any fecal incontinence. This clinical presentation leans towards a small bowel origin rather than colitis, although definitive determination between the two would require further evaluation.

There are many possible organisms that might have caused this case of travelers' diarrhea. Here are the classics:

Enterotoxigenic E. coli (ETEC). This is the most common cause of traveler's diarrhea and can cause watery diarrhea. It's often acquired through the consumption of contaminated food or water.

Don't confuse it with Enterohemorrhagic *E. colitis* (EHEC), especially the famous 0157:H7 serotype, which causes bloody diarrhea and colitis. ETEC is noninvasive, whereas EHEC is invasive.

Enteroaggregative E. coli (EAEC). Speaking for ourselves, we're remiss to admit that we don't think much about this pathogen because ETEC is such a prevalent cause of traveler's diarreha. However, EAEC follows closely behind ETEC as a top cause of traveler's diarrhea and is often attributed to the particularly watery forms of diarrhea.

Shigella. This bacterium can cause bloody diarrhea (i.e., dysentery), fever, and stomach cramps, often spread through direct contact with bacteria in feces. Note, however, that it most often presents as just watery diarrhea without dysentery.

Campylobacter jejuni. This bacterium can cause watery or bloody diarrhea and is commonly associated with consuming under-cooked poultry or contaminated water.

Norovirus. A highly contagious virus that can cause acute onset of vomiting and watery diarrhea. It's often spread through contaminated food or water, as well as person-to-person contact. This is the one that you hear about causing outbreaks on cruise ships.

Salmonella species. These bacteria can cause diarrhea, fever, and abdominal cramps, often after consumption of contaminated meat, poultry, eggs, or produce.

Giardia lamblia. A protozoan parasite that can cause giardiasis, classically leading to foul-smelling (isn't all stool foul-smelling, though?), fatty diarrhea (i.e., steatorrhea). It's usually acquired through drinking contaminated water, such as campers drinking from streams. Not fun.

Cryptosporidium. Another protozoan parasite that can cause watery diarrhea, acquired through contaminated water, including swimming pools and water parks.

While these pathogens are among the most common, the actual cause of diarrhea in travelers can vary and depends on specific exposures and individual susceptibility. Food and water contamination are known to be the source of these infections, although risk reduction through dietary precautions and hygiene don't work as well as we'd like, mainly because the ubiquitous nature and small innocuous that can cause infection.

In the meantime, we can't yet know for sure what is causing the diarrheal illness in this patient. Is stool testing warranted? Most cases of travel-associated acute diarrhea don't need specific investigation as they can be emprically treated with highly effective antibiotics to shorten the duration of illness from a 3-5 day illness to less than

24 hours in most cases. The guidelines instead underscore the potential benefits of appropriate diagnostic testing in cases of severe diarrhea and/or dysentery, in those who those who have failed first line therapy, and among those may live in a congregate setting.

Here's a distilled summary on stool testing:

Advancements in Diagnostics. Traditional methods like bacterial culture and microscopy are time-consuming and have limitations. Newer molecular diagnostic techniques, however, offer rapid, sensitive, and simultaneous detection of a wide range of pathogens, which can enhance the management of diarrheal diseases. These molecular tests outperform older methods in identifying causes of diarrhea and can provide results quickly.

Considerations for Testing. The decision to test should consider the clinical context, such as exposure history and symptom severity, rather than relying solely on traditional indicators like fecal leukocytes. Molecular diagnostics have broadened the range of detectable pathogens but also raised issues of interpreting the clinical significance of detected organisms due to the possibility of identifying non-viable or non-pathogenic levels of microbes.

Limitations and Challenges. Despite their sensitivity, molecular tests can miss new pathogens not included in their panels and cannot distinguish between live and dead organisms. This could lead to challenges in identifying the true cause of illness and understanding the clinical relevance of mixed infections.

Role of Bacterial Culture. While molecular diagnostics are advancing, bacterial culture remains relevant for public health surveillance and understanding antimicrobial resistance patterns. The shift towards culture-independent testing doesn't eliminate the need for traditional methods in certain scenarios, like detecting new diarrheal disease causes or conducting antimicrobial susceptibility testing in outbreak situations.

That said, the guidelines also indicate that empirical treatment with antibiotics generally remains effective for most patients. The low failure rate of empirical antimicrobial therapy suggests that, outside of outbreak settings, specific antimicrobial susceptibility testing may not be necessary for individual patient care.

In any event, wish we could be a little clearer with how best to answer the testing question, but the guidelines are nuanced on that point.

But what about treatment? How best to proceed, and with what antibiotic? The ACG guidelines provide a helpful algorithm to guide next steps (**Figure 2.5**).

The first question in the algorithm is whether the diarrhea is watery or more dysentery-like with bloody stools. In this case, it's the former. Next, they ask if this is a mild illness or a moderate-to-severe illness, where the latter suggests some level of disability or impact on functional status or activities due to the illness. In this case, the patient said the diarrhea is affecting her ability to take care of her young children at home. Next, the algorithm asks whether there are travel-associated symptoms. Here, it's travel related. So, following along, the guidelines next indicate to start antibiotic therapy. You'll notice that it says nothing about whether to test the stool, suggesting that empiric antibiotics are appropriate. Given the travel to Surat, India (which is incidentally known for its delicious, spicy street food and also happens to be the city where one of the authors of this book was born), this patient would be best served to take azithromycin to cover fluoroquinolone-resistant *Campylobacter* or resistant ETEC.

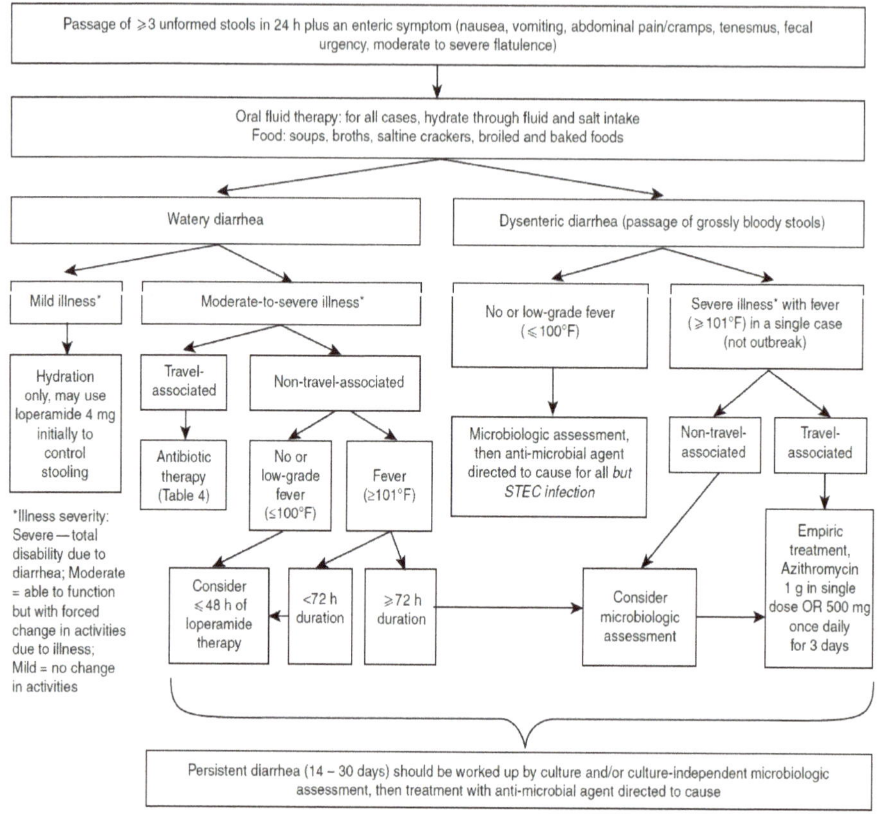

Note, however, that in the absence of travel-related diarrhea, the guidelines do not recommend empiric antibiotics. That's a key distinction. In the case of community-acquired diarrhea, the initial questions focus more on how severe the illness appears, based on the level and duration of fever. If there is a persistent fever for 72 hours or more, then microbiological assessments are warranted to guide antibiotic decision-making (again, check out the algorithm to see these details).

But this is a case of traveler's diarrhea, so empiric antibiotics are indicated. Here is a list of acceptable antibiotics per the guidelines:

Table 2.6. *Acute diarrhea antibiotic regimens.*[80]

Antibiotic[a]	Dose	Treatment duration
Levofloxacin	500 mg by mouth	Single dose[b] or 3-day course
Ciprofloxacin	750 mg by mouth or	Single dose[b]
	500 mg by mouth	3-day course
Ofloxacin	400 mg by mouth	Single dose[b] or 3-day course
Azithromycin[c,d]	1,000 mg by mouth or	Single dose[b]
	500 mg by mouth	3-day course[d]
Rifaximin[e]	200 mg by mouth t.i.d.	3-days

[a]Antibiotic regimens may be combined with loperamide, 4 mg first dose, and then 2 mg dose after each loose stool, not to exceed 16 mg in a 24-h period.
[b]If symptoms are not resolved after 24 h, complete a 3-day course of antibiotics.
[c]Use empirically as first line in Southeast Asia and India to cover fluoroquinolone-resistant *Camplyobacter* or in other geographical areas if *Camplyobacter* or resistant Enterotoxigenic *Escherichia coli* are suspected.
[d]Preferred regiment for dysentery or febrile diarrhea.
[e]Do not use if clinical suspicion for *Camplyobacter Salmonella, Shigella*, or other causes of invasive diarrhea.

Here are key takeaways about treating traveler's diarrhea:

- Combining an antibiotic with loperamide further shortens the illness duration, offering quicker relief from symptoms. In the past, there was concern that using loperamide could worsen outcomes, but that has not been

Yep, it's generally okay to use loperamide in acute traveler's diarrhea

borne out and it's okay to use loperamide unless there is concern for toxicity.

- Azithromycin has shown comparable efficacy to fluoroquinolones in several randomized controlled trials, with specific effectiveness against fluoroquinolone-resistant *Campylobacter* and a broader range of pathogens including *Shigella* and non-invasive diarrheagenic *E. coli*.

- The non-absorbable antibiotic rifaximin is effective against diarrheagenic *E. coli*, the most common pathogen in the Western Hemisphere, without showing significant differences in cure rates compared to ciprofloxacin in studies.

- There are concerns about complicating enteric diseases caused by specific pathogens like Shiga-like toxin-producing *E. coli* and non-typhoidal *Salmonella* strains due to potential adverse effects such as increasing the risk of hemolytic uremic syndrome or prolonging pathogen carriage.

- Antibiotic treatment can alter gut microbiota, potentially leading to *C. difficile*-associated diarrhea or facilitating colonization by resistant bacteria, especially among travelers who self-medicate with antibiotics.

The guidelines emphasize the importance of selecting appropriate antibiotic therapy based on the likely pathogens, local resistance patterns, and specific patient factors, while also considering the potential impacts of antibiotic use on microbial resistance and the individual's microbiota.

If you're dealing with non-severe, non-cholera-like diarrhea, you should probably skip the antibiotics. The game plan here usually includes non-antibiotic anti-diarrheals that cut down on bathroom trips. Antisecretory meds like bismuth subsalicylate can help get to the root of the problem by tackling the excessive intestinal secretions behind watery diarrhea. Bismuth can dial down the number of trips to the bathroom by around 40%.

Okay, that does it for the chapter on bugs. Let's see how much you learned.

GI Infections Guidelines Quiz

1. Which duo of scientists is credited with the discovery of *H. pylori* and its role in gastritis and peptic ulcer disease?

    a) Robert Koch and Louis Pasteur
    b) Alexander Fleming and Howard Florey
    c) Jonas Salk and Albert Sabin
    d) Barry Marshall and Robin Warren
    e) Tom and Jerry

2. What proportion of the North American population is estimated to harbor *H. pylori*?

    a) 10%-20%

    b) 20%-30%

    c) 30%-40%

    d) 40%-50%

3. Which of the following statements is true regarding the epidemiology of *H. pylori* infection?

    a) *H. pylori* is more common in developed countries compared to developing countries

    b) *H. pylori* rates decrease with age

    c) *H. pylori* is a rare cause of dyspepsia.

    d) *H. pylori* infection is more prevalent in lower socioeconomic groups and crowded living conditions.

4. *H. pylori* "test and treat" means:

   a) Test for *H. pylori,* and then hem and haw about whether to treat it should the test come back positive.

   b) Test for *H. pylori,* and then offer treatment if the test is positive.

5. All of the following are indications to test and treat for *H. pylori* infection except:

   a) Patients with a history of peptic ulcer disease

   b) Individuals with functional dyspepsia

   c) Patients with autoimmune gastritis

   d) Patients with acid reflux disease and erosive esophagitis

   e) Patients with idiopathic thrombocytopenic purpura (ITP)

6. A 50-year-old man presents with epigastric pain and occasional nausea that has persisted for several weeks. He reports that the pain often worsens after meals. He has no significant past medical history and does not take any regular medications. An upper endoscopy reveals a peptic ulcer in the duodenum. A biopsy and subsequent testing confirm the presence of *H. pylori* infection. According to the ACG guidelines, which of the following is the preferred first-line therapy?

   a) Triple therapy with a PPI, clarithromycin, and amoxicillin

   b) Bismuth quadruple therapy (BQT)

   c) Sequential therapy with a PPI and antibiotics

   d) High-dose dual therapy with a PPI and amoxicillin

7. Which of the following statements about BQT for *H. pylori* infection is true?

   a) BQT includes a bismuth salt, metronidazole, doxycycline, and a PPI.

   b) H2 receptor antagonists are recommended by ACG guidelines for use in BQT.

   c) BQT should always be prescribed for 14 days

   d) BQT is less effective than PPI-clarithromycin triple therapy in the presence of clarithromycin resistance.

8. Which of the following statements about vonoprazan, a potassium competitive acid blocker (PCAB), is true regarding its use in treating *H. pylori* infection?

   a) Vonoprazan must be taken with meals to ensure efficacy.

   b) Vonoprazan-based therapy requires antibiotic resistance testing before initiation.

   c) Vonoprazan maintains a higher intragastric pH than traditional PPIs, enhancing antibiotic efficacy.

   d) Vonoprazan is ineffective against clarithromycin-resistant strains of *H. pylori*.

9. According to the ACG guidelines, which of the following statements is true regarding the use of clarithromycin and levofloxacin in the treatment of *H. pylori* infection?

   a) Clarithromycin and levofloxacin should be used as first-line treatments without the need for susceptibility testing.

   b) Clarithromycin should only be used if the *H. pylori* strain is con-firmed to be sensitive to it.

   c) Levofloxacin is recommended due to its lower side effect profile compared to other antibiotics.

   d) Clarithromycin-based regimens should be preferred over alternatives like amoxicillin or tetracycline.

10. According to the ACG guidelines, how should the eradication of *H. pylori* be confirmed after treatment?

a) Using serology tests immediately after treatment completion

b) Performing a urea breath test, fecal antigen test, or gastric biopsy at least 4 weeks after treatment

c) Continuously using acid blockers like PPIs up to the day of testing

d) Testing for eradication immediately after the last dose of antibiotics

11. In which of the following circumstances is it acceptable to treat for *H. pylori* and not confirm cure?

a) Dyspepsia

b) Peptic ulcer bleed

c) MALT lymphoma

d) Idiopathic thrombocytopenic purpura (ITP)

e) It is never acceptable to treat *H. pylori* without confirming cure

12. A 55-year-old man with a history of peptic ulcer disease was treated for *H. pylori* infection. His initial regimen was a PPI-clarithromycin triple therapy, but follow-up testing showed persistent infection. He has no known allergies. What is the most appropriate next step in managing his *H. pylori* infection?

a) Repeat PPI-clarithromycin triple therapy

b) Optimized BQT

c) High-dose PPI or PCAB dual therapy

d) Amoxicillin and metronidazole combination therapy

13. A 45-year-old woman with a penicillin allergy has a history of persistent *H. pylori* infection. She was previously treated with a non-optimized BQT but remains infected. What is the most appropriate salvage regimen for her condition?

a) Repeat non-optimized BQT

b) PPI-clarithromycin triple therapy

c) High-dose PPI or PCAB dual therapy

d) Optimized BQT

14. A 60-year-old man with a history of persistent *H. pylori* infection has undergone antibiotic susceptibility testing. The results show that the strain is clarithromycin-sensitive and levofloxacin-resistant. What is the most appropriate salvage regimen for his *H. pylori* infection according to the ACG guidelines?

a) Clarithromycin triple therapy

b) Levofloxacin triple therapy

c) High-dose PPI or PCAB dual therapy

d) Optimized BQT

15. A 48-year-old woman with persistent *H. pylori* infection undergoes susceptibility testing. The results show that the strain is resistant to both clarithromycin and levofloxacin. What is the most appropriate salvage regimen?

a) Clarithromycin triple therapy

b) Levofloxacin triple therapy

c) Optimized BQT

d) Amoxicillin and metronidazole combination therapy

16. In which of the following scenarios should testing for *C. difficile* be considered?

a) A patient with 2 loose stools per day for 1 week

b) A patient experiencing new, unexplained diarrhea with at least 3 loose stools per day

c) A patient with no symptoms but a history of recent antibiotic use

d) Routine testing for all patients upon hospital admission

17. A 70-year-old woman with a history of recent hospitalization for pneumonia presents with 2 loose stools per day for the past 4 days. She is otherwise asymptomatic and has no fever or abdominal pain. Her medical history includes type 2 diabetes and chronic kidney disease. Given her recent antibiotic use and hospitalization, CDI is suspected. Initial testing with a NAAT returns positive. Then, a toxin EIA is performed and returns negative. Based on the diagnostic algorithm, what is the appropriate interpretation and next step for this patient's management?

a) The patient has a confirmed CDI and should be treated accordingly

b) The patient is likely colonized with *C. difficile* but does not have an active infection

c) Perform a repeat NAAT to confirm the initial result

d) Empirically treat the patient with antibiotics for CDI

18. Why is it necessary to follow up a positive GDH or NAAT with a toxin EIA test when diagnosing CDI?

a) The GDH and NAAT tests have a high false-negative rate

b) Unlike the EIA, the GDH and NAAT tests cannot distinguish between toxigenic and non-toxigenic strains of *C. difficile*

c) The GDH and NAAT tests are not sensitive enough to detect CDI.

d) The GDH and NAAT tests are only used to monitor treatment response.

19. What is the white blood cell threshold for categorizing a *C. difficile* infection as severe?

    a) 10,000 cells/mL

    b) 15,000 cells/mL

    c) 20,000 cells/mL

    d) 25,000 cells/mL

20. According to the latest ACG guidelines, which of the following is now recommended as the primary treatment for non-severe *C. difficile* infection?

    a) Metronidazole

    b) Vancomycin or fidaxomicin

    c) Rifaximin

    d) Ciprofloxacin

21. Why is fidaxomicin considered a favorable option for treating *C. difficile* despite its higher cost?

    a) It is more effective against a broader range of bacteria

    b) It has lower recurrence rates and is directed specifically at *C. difficile*

    c) It is easier to administer than vancomycin

    d) It is less likely to cause side effects compared to other antibiotics

22. In which scenario might metronidazole still be considered a viable first-line treatment option for non-severe CDI?

    a) For older patients with multiple comorbidities

    b) For younger, healthier outpatients who are concerned about cost

    c) For patients with severe CDI

    d) For patients who have failed vancomycin therapy

23. What is a major reason why the ACG guidelines do not currently recommend rifaximin for routine first-line therapy of CDI?

a) High resistance rates

b) Low effectiveness compared to other antibiotics

c) High cost

d) Lack of availability

24. How does fidaxomicin's effect on the microbiome compare to that of vancomycin in the treatment of CDI?

a) Fidaxomicin is more likely to disrupt the microbiome than vancomycin

b) Fidaxomicin maintains a more diverse microbiome by not affecting other commensals as much as vancomycin.

c) Vancomycin is more selective for *C. difficile* than fidaxomicin.

d) Both fidaxomicin and vancomycin have similar effects on the microbiome.

25. Why is metronidazole no longer recommended as a first-line treatment for severe CDI?

a) It has higher recurrence rates compared to vancomycin.

b) It is less effective and associated with adverse outcomes such as extended hospitalization and increased acute kidney injury.

c) It is more expensive than vancomycin and fidaxomicin.

d) It has significant drug-drug interactions compared to vancomycin.

26. What did a head-to-head comparison of vancomycin dosing reveal about the effectiveness of 125 mg versus 500 mg in treating severe CDI?

a) The 500 mg dose is significantly more effective.

b) The 125 mg dose is significantly more effective.

c) Both doses are equally effective.

d) Neither dose is effective in treating severe CDI.

27. What is the primary advantage of fidaxomicin over vancomycin in the treatment of CDI?

a) Lower cost

b) Higher initial cure rates

c) Lower recurrence rates

d) Fewer side effects

28. What role does FMT play in the treatment of severe and fulminant CDI?

a) FMT is a first-line treatment for all cases of CDI.

b) FMT is not recommended for severe CDI.

c) FMT is used for severe and fulminant CDI that doesn't respond to standard therapies.

d) FMT is primarily used to treat mild cases of CDI.

29. What is a significant benefit of FMT for patients with severe and fulminant CDI?

a) It eliminates the need for antibiotic therapy.

b) It reduces the need for colectomy and lowers the incidence of CDI-related sepsis.

c) It replaces the need for vancomycin and fidaxomicin.

d) It has no effect on the overall survival rates of critically ill patients.

30. What is the recommended follow-up treatment for patients who improve enough to be discharged but still have pseudomembranes?

a) Discontinue all antibiotics immediately

b) Continue oral vancomycin or fidaxomicin at home, followed by an outpatient FMT

c) Start a new course of metronidazole

d) Monitor without any further treatment

31. How is clinical improvement monitored after FMT for severe and fulminant CDI?

a) By checking stool consistency and frequency, the absence of pseudomembranes, and normalized inflammatory markers like white blood cell count and CRP levels

b) By performing daily colonoscopies

c) By stopping all medications and observing the patient's symptoms

d) By relying on patient-reported symptom relief

32. Which of the following is true about use of FMT for patients with recurrent *C. difficile* infection (rCDI)?

a) It only addresses the immediate infection without affecting recurrence rates

b) It has a high success rate in reducing the likelihood of recurrence

c) It is less effective than traditional antibiotics for long-term treatment

d) It is primarily used as a last resort treatment option after repeated rounds of antibiotics have failed

33. Which of the following is a common symptom associated with FMT?

    a) Severe allergic reaction

    b) Abdominal discomfort or bloating

    c) Persistent diarrhea

    d) Chronic fatigue

34. What alternative treatment strategy can be used for managing rCDI in patients who are not eligible for FMT or have relapsed post-FMT?

    a) Long-term suppressive oral vancomycin

    b) Intravenous antibiotics

    c) Surgical intervention

    d) High-dose corticosteroids

35. What does the ACG guideline emphasize about FMT in the treatment of rCDI?

    a) FMT should only be used as a last resort treatment

    b) FMT is a significant advancement in treating rCDI with a high success rate

    c) FMT is less effective and more risky compared to traditional antibiotics

    d) FMT is only recommended for mild cases of CDI

36. A 65-year-old man with a long history of GERD controlled by PPIs develops CDI. What should be considered regarding the continuation of PPI therapy in this patient?

   a) Discontinue PPI therapy immediately due to the high risk of CDI

   b) Continue PPI therapy if there are valid medical reasons, as the benefits outweigh the slight risk of CDI

   c) Switch from PPI therapy to H2 receptor antagonists to eliminate CDI risk

   d) Continue PPI therapy only if no other risk factors for CDI are present

37. A 45-year-old man with a history of ulcerative colitis, previously well-controlled on infliximab, presents with new-onset bloody diarrhea and significant weight loss. He does not report use of NSAIDs, recent travel, dietary changes, or antibiotic use. Stool tests return positive for *C. difficile*. Colonoscopy reveals continuous colonic inflammation without pseudomembranes. What is the most appropriate next step in managing this patient?

   a) Discontinue infliximab and start a 10-day course of vancomycin 125mg by mouth 4 times daily (PO QID)

   b) Continue infliximab and start a minimum 14-day course of vancomycin 125mg PO QID

   c) Start fidaxomicin and hold infliximab until symptoms resolve

   d) Perform fecal microbiota transplant (FMT) immediately

38. What is the recommended duration of vancomycin therapy for a patient with ulcerative colitis and a confirmed CDI?

   a) 5 days

   b) 10 days

   c) A minimum of 14 days

   d) 21 days

39. What is the likelihood of IBD patients presenting with pseudomembranes on endoscopy when they have CDI?

a) Very high, nearly 100%

b) Moderate, around 50%

c) Low, they seldom present with pseudomembranes

d) Variable, depending on the severity of CDI

40. What is the success rate of FMT in eradicating CDI in patients
with IBD?

a) 50%

b) 65%

c) 90%

d) 100%

41. What proportion of IBD patients may experience worse symptoms post-FMT, despite its effectiveness in clearing CDI?

a) 0%-5%

b) 7%-25%

c) 30%-50%

d) 60%-75%

42. What is the most common cause of traveler's diarrhea in the
United States?

a) *Salmonella*

b) *Shigella*

c) *Escherichia coli*

d) *Campylobacter*

43. A 30-year-old woman presents to the clinic with a 2-week history of persistent diarrhea, abdominal cramping, bloating, and foul-smelling, greasy stools. She reports that her symptoms began shortly after returning from a hiking trip in the mountains, where she drank water from natural streams without using any purification methods. She does not report any fever, blood in the stool, or recent antibiotic use. Physical examination reveals mild abdominal tenderness but no significant findings. What is the most likely diagnosis for this patient?

a) Viral gastroenteritis

b) Cryptosporidiosis

c) Giardiasis

d) Shigella

e) Norovirus

44. A 45-year-old man presents to the clinic with a 2-day history of watery diarrhea, experiencing more than 3 unformed stools per day. He also reports mild nausea and abdominal cramping but no vomiting, fever, or blood in the stool. He has no significant past medical history and has not recently traveled. On exam, he appears well-hydrated with mild abdominal tenderness. What is the most appropriate initial management for this patient?

a) Prescribe antibiotics immediately

b) Advise oral fluid therapy and over-the-counter loperamide

c) Order a stool culture

d) Admit to the hospital for intravenous fluids

45. A 32-year-old woman presents to the ED with a 3-day history of severe abdominal pain, vomiting, and bloody diarrhea after returning from a trip to Mexico. She has had more than 10 episodes of diarrhea per day and reports a fever of 101.5°F. On examination, she appears dehydrated, with a temperature of 102°F, tachycardia, and significant abdominal tenderness. What is the most appropriate next step in managing this patient?

a) Administer intravenous fluids and observe

b) Start empirical antibiotic therapy and obtain stool cultures

c) Recommend oral fluid therapy and bed rest at home

d) Prescribe loperamide and send the patient home

GI Infections Guidelines Quiz Answers

1.	D		24.	B
2.	C		25.	B
3.	D		26.	C
4.	B		27.	C
5.	D		28.	C
6.	B		29.	B
7.	C		30.	B
8.	C		31.	A
9.	B		32.	B
10.	B		33.	B
11.	E		34.	A
12.	B		35.	B
13.	D		36.	B
14.	A		37.	B
15.	C		38.	C
16.	B		39.	C
17.	B		40.	C
18.	B		41.	B
19.	B		42.	C
20.	B		43.	C
21.	B		44.	B
22.	B		45.	B
23.	A			

Chapter Three

WHEN THE RIVER RUNS RED

Deciphering the Dilemmas of GI Bleeding

Let's face it, many of us dreamed of being surgeons. We loved procedures and fixing things with our hands. Maybe you enjoyed your surgery rotation but thought, "Man, they sure get up early, and I also like thinking through stuff." GI offers that perfect balance between internal medicine and surgery.

Nowhere is that more evident than with GI bleeding. While our medicine colleagues might get queasy at the sight of a pumping vessel, we run towards it, scope in hand, ready to save lives. It's that surgeon's instinct in us.

In this chapter, we'll dive into the ACG guidelines on GI bleeding. We'll cover managing peptic ulcer hemorrhage, guidelines on lower GI bleeding and colon ischemia, and the safe use of anticoagulants and antiplatelet drugs during acute GI bleeding. This is critical stuff: the information you need for those 3:00 AM emergency calls. Let's jump right in with ulcer bleeding!

Case 3.1: GI Bleeder in the ED

A 53-year-old tennis enthusiast presents to the ED with melena for the past 24 hours. He takes a statin for hyperlipidemia and naproxen for tennis elbow due to overhitting his forehand, as he was trying to play like Roger Federer. He has no other significant medical history. He feels well without chest pain, lightheadedness, or fatigue.

On examination, his blood pressure is 112/65; heart rate 82 bpm. He looks well, and his abdomen is soft and non-tender, not distended. A rectal exam reveals melenic stool.

Lab results: Hgb 13.4; BUN 16; creatinine 0.9; WBC 6.1; Platelets 230; albumin 4.1; total bilirubin 0.7; International Normalized Ratio (INR) 1.0.

You are consulted by the attending to consider admission to the hos-pital and asked for an inpatient upper endoscopy due to "melanotic" stool.

Know your guidelines!

What is the next most appropriate step?

Case 3.1: What do the guidelines say?

Source: ACG 2021 Upper GI and Ulcer Bleeding Guideline[81]

This is a common scenario faced by GI providers. So, what are you going to tell the ED attending? She wanted you to admit the patient for upper endoscopy. Is that necessary? What do the guidelines recommend? Let's first take a look at some of the evidence that formed the guidelines.

Although it's straightforward to conclude that an active GI bleeder needs to be admitted, it can be harder to tell whether to admit patients with only subtle signs of bleeding. When is it safe to discharge someone straight from the ED? Lucky for us, the ACG guidelines have clear advice on this, and it comes down to understanding the Glasgow-Blatchford score (GBS; **Table 3.1**).[82]

The GBS is an essential risk assessment tool that every GI provider should have at their fingertips.[83] It's based on 8 easily obtainable risk factors at presentation. Each factor is assigned a score, and the total GBS is the sum of these individual scores. Patients with a GBS of 0 or 1 are at very low risk, with a ≤1% chance of requiring hospital-based interventions such as transfusions, hemostatic procedures, or facing mortality. This means a patient with a GBS of 0 or 1 has a 99% sensitivity, indicating that only 1 out of 100 patients will need hospital-based care or experience a severe outcome. High sensitivity is crucial because it minimizes false negatives, ensuring that we don't send patients home only to have them return with complications. Conversely, patients showing signs of significant GI bleeding or having hepatic or cardiac diseases should be admitted for further evaluation and management. Essentially, any patient with a GBS of 2 or higher should be admitted for inpatient care.

Table 3.1. *Glasgow-Blatchford Score*[82]

Risk factors at admission	Factor Score
Blood urea nitrogen (mg/dL)	
18.2 to <22.4	2
22.4 to <28.0	3
28.0 to <70.0	4
≥70.0	6
Hemoglobin (g/dL)	
12.0 to <13.0 (men); 10.0 to <12.0 (women)	1
10.0 to <12.0 (men)	3
<10.0	6
Systolic blood pressure (mm Hg)	
100-109	1
90-99	2
<90	3
Heart rate (beats per minute)	
≥100	1
Melana	1
Syncope	2
Hepatic disease[a]	2
Cardiac failure[a]	2
[a]Hepatic disease and cardiac failure were not defined in the original report of the Glasgow-Blatchford score. One more recent study defined hepatic disease as known history, or clinical and laboratory evidence, of chronic or acute liver disease and cardiac failure as known history, or clinical and echocardiographic evidence, of cardiac failure.[83]	

If you calculate the GBS for the patient in the vignette, you'll find that his total GBS is 1, since melena is his only accumulated point from the risk factors. Based on this evidence, you can confidently tell the ED attending that the patient can be safely discharged and arrange for outpatient followup. Additionally, it's worth educating the ED attending on the proper terminology. "Melanotic" describes darker skin and tissue pigmentation, which is more appropriate for dermatologic conditions. On the other hand, "melenic" is the correct term to describe dark, tarry stool. This distinction is important, though hopefully, you won't encounter the rare case of melanoma defecation, as melanoma can occasionally metastasize to the GI tract.

You should counsel the patient to lay off the naproxen and/or go easy on the forehand. After all, there is only one Roger Federer, the GOAT (Greatest-Of-All-Time) of men's tennis, who has an incredible forehand, which is extremely diffi-cult to emulate (author B.S. wishes to emphasize that this comment is from author H.K., although B.S. has no particular issues with Roger Federer). At any rate, there will be significant cost savings for the patient and the healthcare system by avoiding hospitalization in this case.

Of note, this does not mean you should instruct every GI bleed pa-tient with a GBS of 0 or 1 to head straight home. Every patient needs to be judged on a case-by-case basis. For example, are there other fac-tors that are not covered in the GBS that might trigger a decision to admit, such as advanced age or other significant health-related prob-lems? Is there adequate social support and access to medical care af-ter discharge to adequately comply with outpatient follow-up? If so, then hospital admission may be the better part of valor.

Case 3.2: Stat EGD

A 71-year-old woman presents to the ED due to black, tarry stools for the past 12 hours accompanied by marked fatigue. She has been taking diclofenac for low back pain for the past 3 weeks. There has been no vomiting, abdominal pain, chest pain or syncope. She has only been hospitalized twice in her lifetime, once for acute appendicitis and once for childbirth. She reports feeling well when she went hiking 2 days ago. She had felt well 2 days ago but now has marked fatigue.

On physical examination: blood pressure (BP) 86/54, heart rate (HR) 108, Temp 98.10 F. Her abdomen is soft and not tender. There is no stool in the rectal vault.

Laboratory tests: Hgb 7.6; BUN 33; Platelets 234; ALT 14; total bilirubin 0.9; INR 1.0

You're the on-call GI consultant for the ED (sorry about that). The ED attending asks you a series of questions about managing this patient:

1. *Should we start transfusion?*

2. *Should we place nasogastric (NG) tube to obtain an aspirate?*

3. *Should we start prokinetic therapy?*

4. *Should we start PPI therapy?*

5. *Can you do a stat EGD?*

Know your guidelines!

How should you address these questions?

Case 3.2: What do the guidelines say?

Source: ACG 2021 Upper GI and Ulcer Bleeding Guideline[81]

The ED has barraged you with a bunch of questions here. They just need some help and that is why we are consultants. Let's tackle one query at a time.

Transfusion. Unless you're dealing with massive exsanguination, it's crucial not to indiscriminately transfuse patients with blood products. Recent international guidelines from the Association for the Advancement of Blood & Biotherapies recommend a restrictive transfusion strategy for most hospitalized adult patients, including critically ill patients who are hemodynamically stable, suggesting transfusion when hemoglobin concentration drops below 7 g/dL.[84] For patients undergoing cardiac surgery, a threshold of 7.5 g/dL can be considered, and for those undergoing orthopedic surgery or with pre-existing cardiovascular disease, a threshold of 8 g/dL is recommended. A significant part of the evidence supporting these guidelines comes from a randomized, controlled trial in Barcelona, which found a significant mortality benefit over 45 days when comparing a restrictive transfusion threshold of 7 g/dL to a more liberal policy of 9 g/dL (5% vs 9% mortality, respectively; $P=0.02$).[85] The Kaplan-Meier survival curve from the study is noted in **Figure 3.1.**

Moreover, the study found increased further bleeding in the liberal-strategy group (16%) compared to the restrictive-strategy group (10%, $P=0.01$). With this background, let's return to our patient in the ED. Should she be transfused? Recall that she presented with hypotension, tachycardia, and anemia with a hemoglobin of 7.6. Her hemoglobin is likely to drop further after volume resuscitation and equilibration, even without additional bleeding. Therefore, she should receive packed red blood cells now. Don't sit on the hemoglobin value.

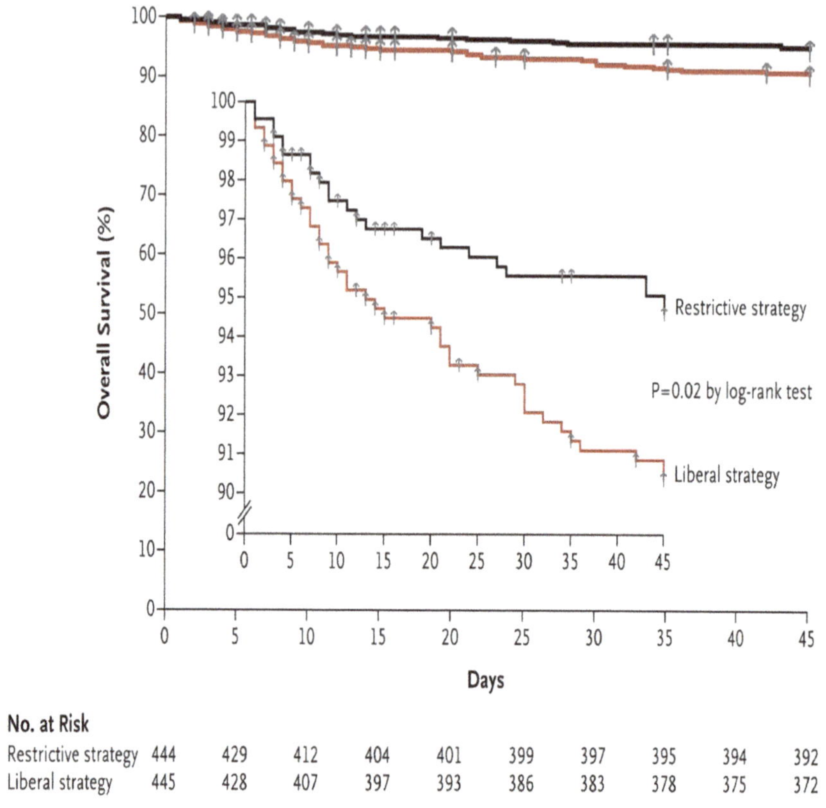

Figure 3.1. *Survival, according to transfusion strategy.*[85]

Is there a specific hemoglobin number that one should target for a bleeding and hypotensive patient? Well, not really. Since clinical situations vary with different degrees of intravascular volume depletion and hemodynamic instability, there is no specific target hemoglobin number as a goal for most patients. Just know that the ACG guidelines suggest that you should not wait for the hemoglobin to fall below 7 g/dL before transfusing a bleeding patient with hypotension. But what if our patient had pre-existing cardiovascular disease? In such a case with a bleeding, hypotensive patient with pre-existing cardiovascular disease, you don't want it to get below 8 g/dL. When

Transfuse for hgb < 8 g/dL if hypotensive or pre-existing CV disease. Don't wait for it drop further with equilibration after volume resuscitation!

you know it's going to drop, it is reasonable for transfusion at higher values if clinically indicated. Suffice it to say that you need to stay on top of these patients and their hemoglobin.

Nasogastric tube aspiration. How about requesting a nasogastric (NG) tube placement with aspiration and lavage for blood prior to endoscopy? This is the old-school GI consultant delay tactic. Both of us learned to do this as fellows, but in retrospect, we're not sure why NG lavage was so vital (Hint: it wasn't). In reality, there is little need for this request. A randomized trial found that NG tube placement didn't accurately predict high-risk endoscopic lesions, even when coffee grounds or red blood were noted in the aspirate compared to the group without NG tube placement. There was no difference in rebleeding rates or mortality. In fact, 34% of patients in the NG aspirate group experienced pain, nasal bleeding, or failed NG tube placement.[86] So, it doesn't help, is not accurate, and doesn't usually affect management. Remember, adequately resuscitating the patient is by far the most important task before endoscopy. That said, we have both seen the occasional situation where NG lavage was useful, like a lower GI bleed where everyone assumes it's from the colon but turns out the stomach or duodenum is bleeding. Or, the patient who is hypotensive with no signs of obvious bleeding, and then the NG lavage comes back positive. So, this can have a useful role on rare occasions.

> No need to routinely request NG tube placement for GI bleeders

Prokinetics. How about prokinetics prior to EGD? It makes sense, doesn't it? You want to see what you're doing. Thus, prokinetic agents can ideally help push the blood further downstream for better visualization. Although there's no evidence showing an improvement in mortality or rebleeding, a systematic review noted that erythromycin decreased length of stay and the need for a second-look endoscopy.[87] This translated to an economic benefit with reduced costs for a shorter hospital course.

> Erythromycin is recommended prior to EGD in UGI bleeding patients

What about metoclopramide? Well, it hasn't generated as much enthusiasm. An initial meta-analysis[88] and further data noted that metoclopramide did not convincingly improve mucosal visualization[89] or reduce the need for repeat endoscopy.[90] Moreover, a recent Thai randomized controlled trial also found no significant improvement in endoscopic visualization with metoclopramide compared with placebo (77% vs 62%).[91] The study was small (62 total subjects) with insignificant trends that suggested a larger study might potentially show some benefit of metoclopramide. Interestingly, a large multi-center, randomized, double-blind, controlled trial[92] also from Thailand was recently published with 300 patients comparing metoclopramide with placebo in patients with acute upper GI bleeding. This study only showed minimal improvement in endoscopic mucosal visualization in the metoclopramide group, but no difference in the rate of repeat EGD (3.5% vs 4.3%) or length of stay (1.78 days vs 1.84 days) compared to placebo. Thus, for now, erythromycin remains the prokinetic of choice and is recommended before endoscopy in patients with an upper GI bleed. It's important to recall that intravenous erythromycin can prolong the QT interval, especially with rapid infusion.

The guidelines recommend a 250 mg infusion of erythromycin 20 to 90 minutes before endoscopy to decrease the need for a second-look endoscopy and reduce hospital stay. Since erythromycin is a cytochrome P450 3A inhibitor, don't forget to look out for drug-drug interactions (we all do a medication reconciliation on each consult anyway, right?) and monitor for the potential of QT prolongation.

Pre-endoscopic PPIs. It seems like intravenous PPIs are started as soon as patients hit the ED with even a hint of a GI bleed. After all, PPIs significantly increase the gastric pH to help stabilize clots. But is there solid evidence to support their preemptive usage? Not really. There's no scientific verification that pre-endoscopic PPI therapy improves clinical outcomes. Yes, that's correct. There's no evidence showing improvements in hard outcomes like reduction in further bleeding, need for surgery, or mortality. This was confirmed by a well-done randomized controlled trial (RCT) from Hong Kong comparing IV omeprazole with placebo (**Table 3.2**), which showed no difference in further bleeding, death, hospital duration, or the amount of blood transfused.[93] However, there was a reduction in the need for endoscopic therapy in the omeprazole group compared to the placebo group. Interestingly, a meta-analysis conducted by the guideline authors also confirmed a similar reduction of hemostatic treatment at the index endoscopy, suggesting that PPIs may help to decrease high-risk bleeding stigmata.[94]

Moreover, there is a possibility that PPIs could potentially help those who can't get endoscopy (e.g., really sick patients) or if endoscopy is unavailable in the short term. After analyzing the extensive data, the ACG guidelines could not reach a recommendation for or against pre-endoscopic PPI therapy for patients with UGIB. In fact, different guidelines have differing opinions on this. For example, an update[95] summarized a British guideline[96], which did not endorse the use of PPIs prior to endoscopy since there has been no improvement in clinically relevant endpoints, such as rebleeding, need for surgery, or mortality. Conversely, the European guidelines[97] mention that PPIs can be considered prior to EGD due to downgrading stigmata of recent hemorrhage at the index endoscopy.

That being said, in the combined experience of the authors of this book, we tend to advise for pre-endoscopic PPIs to potentially decrease high-risk stigmata and hopefully make that initial EGD a little smoother. Besides, we are seeing older and sicker patients getting admitted with upper GI bleeding (UGIB), and sometimes they have too many medical issues to scope in a timely manner, if at all. So, if you are taking care of those elderly, ill patients with multiple comorbidities and an UGIB, then empiric PPIs might be useful. In some cases, they may not ever get well enough to scope at all. In the end, it's up to you to decide on a case-by-case basis whether or not to advise PPIs prior to EGD.

Table 3.2. *Randomized trial comparing omeprazole vs placebo prior to EGD for UGIB.*[93]

Outcome	Omeprazole (N=314)	Placebo (N=317)
Hours of infusion before endoscopy, mean ± SD	14.7 ±6.3	15.2 ±6.2
Further bleeding (30 d), n (%)	11 (3.5)	8 (2.5)
Death (30 d), n (%)	8 (2.5)	7 (2.2)
Hospital days, mean ± SD	4.5 ±5.3	4.9 ±5.1
Units of blood transfused, mean ± SD	1.54 ±2.41	1.88 ±3.44
Endoscopic therapy, n (%)	60 (19.1)[a]	90 (28.4)

[a] $P = 0007$ vs placebo.

Timing of Endoscopy. It seems like we are living in an instant gratification society. Everybody wants everything immediately. The ED is asking for a "stat" EGD. Is this necessary? I mean, we're not just technicians who do things on command. We are GI providers, and we think about things before blindly proceeding. This "stat" request is the GI's pet peeve. Well, sometimes faster is not always better. The ACG guidelines recommend that patients admitted for UGIB should get an EGD within 24 hours of presentation. The data on that is pretty straightforward and one of your authors even published his very first paper on this very topic. There is cost-saving when the EGD is performed within 24 hours due to earlier discharge, decreased need for surgery, and a mortality benefit. But what about this request for a "stat" EGD? Is doing it even sooner better?

> EGD should be done within 24 hours of presentation in low risk and high risk patients with UGIB

A large, randomized trial (**Table 3.3**) with over 500 patients who presented with high-risk UGIB for further bleeding or death, defined as a GBS ≥ 12, stratified patients in regard to the timing of EGD in relation to time of the GI consultation: within 6 hours (very early endoscopy) vs within 6-24 hours (early endoscopy).[99] They found that there was no reduction in mortality or rebleeding within 30 days in the very early endoscopy group compared to the early endoscopy group In line with this study, the ACG guideline authors recommended that resuscitation and treatment of other comorbidities should be the first priority rather than jumping straight to endoscopy after the initial GI consult. Sometimes it's worthwhile to remind our colleagues about the basics of resuscitation, including that 2 large bore IVs should be placed in patients with UGIB.

Table 3.3. *Randomized trial comparing timing of EGD in patient with UGIB and GBS $\geq$ 12.*[99]

Outcome	Endoscopy <6 hr (N=258)	Endoscopy 6-24 hr (N=258)
Hours from presentation to endoscopy, mean $\pm$ SD	9.9 $\pm$ 6.1	24.7 $\pm$ 9.0
Further bleeding (30 d), n (%)	28 (10.9)	20 (7.8)
Death (30 d), n (%)	23 (8.9)	17 (6.6)
Hospital days, median (range)	5 (4-9)	5 (3-8)
Units of blood transfused, mean $\pm$ SD	2.4 $\pm$ 2.3	2.4 $\pm$ 2.1
Endoscopic therapy, n (%)	155 (60.1)[a]	125 (48.4)
[a] $P = 0001$ vs endoscopy 6-24 hours.		

Case 3.3: Black diarrhea

A 62-year-old woman presents to the emergency department with "black diarrhea" for the past 2 days, accompanied by lightheadedness and fatigue. In the ED, she is hypotensive with a blood pressure of 98/62 and tachycardic with a heart rate of 108 in sinus rhythm. Her hemoglobin level is 9.3 g/dL. Her abdominal examination is unremarkable. She is resuscitated with intravenous fluids and hemodynamically stabilized. You are consulted and perform an EGD the next morning, which shows the following image (**Figure 3.2**):

Figure 3.2. *Gastric ulcer at the incisura. Image source: J. Andy Tau, MD.*

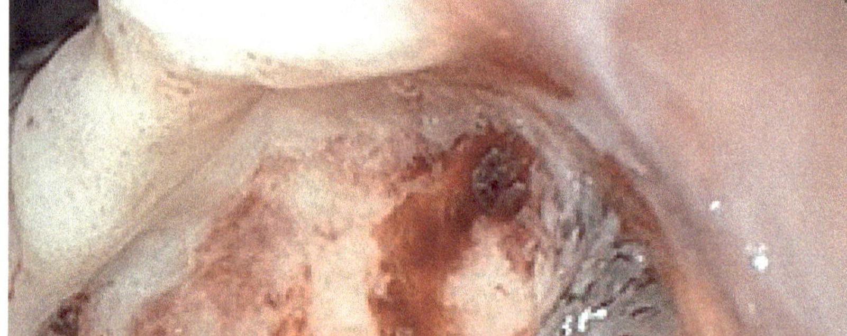

Know your guidelines!

1. What are you going to do during this EGD?

2. Will PPI therapy be beneficial here?

Case 3.3: What do the guidelines say?

Source: ACG 2021 Upper GI and Ulcer Bleeding Guideline[81]

Recognizing the endoscopic stigmata of recent hemorrhage is vital for any GI practitioner. The importance of this knowledge has been ingrained in us since our fellowship days and continues to be crucial during inpatient calls. Not only is identifying these stigmata essential, but understanding the associated risk of rebleeding without endoscopic intervention is equally important. John Forrest and colleagues first described use of early endoscopy on patients admitted for upper GI bleeding in 1974,[100] and their work remains relevant today. **Table 3.4)** is a summary of the rebleeding risks associated with each type of recent hemorrhage stigmata, emphasizing the necessity of timely and effective endoscopic therapy.

Take a closer look at that ulcer image: there's a plump, non-bleeding (at least for now) visible vessel sitting right at 2 o'clock near the ulcer crater rim. So, what's the next step? This is where endoscopic therapy really shines. Numerous studies have demonstrated its effectiveness. A comprehensive meta-analysis[88] found that endoscopic therapy is highly effective for non-bleeding visible vessels, with a Number Needed to Treat (NNT) of 5 compared to placebo. Even more impressive, for active bleeding (defined as active spurting and/or oozing), the NNT is just 2 in favor of endoscopic therapy over placebo. It's no surprise that the guidelines strongly recommend endoscopic therapy for both non-bleeding visible vessels and active bleeding to improve patient outcomes.

So, which specific type of endoscopic hemostatic therapy should you use? The data strongly support thermal contact devices like bipolar electrocoagulation and the heater probe. These tools combine direct pressure on the vessel with electrical energy to achieve hemostasis by effectively welding the culprit artery shut. They are particularly effective for both active bleeding and non-bleeding visible vessels. Given

Table 3.4. *Stigmata of recent hemorrhage and risk of rebleeding without endoscopic therapy.*[101,102]

Stigmata	Forrest Classification	Rebleeding risk	Image of Forrest Classification
Active bleeding	1A (spurting)	55%	1A
	1B (oozing)		1B
Non-bleeding visible vessel	2A	43%	2A
Adherent clot	2B	22%	2B
Flat pigmented spot	2C	10%	2C
Clean ulcer base	3	5%	3

the size of the vessel in the image, make sure to use a larger probe, such as the 10 French bipolar coagulation probe or the 3.2 mm heater probe, especially for larger vessels. The last thing you want is to deal with torrential bleeding from a large vessel that was incompletely cauterized with a smaller probe.

Clips work well too. The use of mechanical clip placement has become more widespread in recent years as the technology has evolved. It's not surprising that there is a relative lack of RCTs comparing clips to placebo since they came around after thermal contact therapy. Although trials comparing clips to thermal contact therapy have shown no major difference, the studies were generally low quality with wide confidence intervals for the treatment effect. Thus, the guideline provides a conditional recommendation for utilizing clips.

Mechanical clip placement has evolved and shown to be an effective hemostatic therapy

Argon plasma coagulation (APC) may help control bleeding ulcers, but the evidence isn't strong enough to firmly recommend its use. While the guidelines do offer a conditional recommendation for APC, employing this modality can be technically challenging due to the need for simultaneous suctioning to reduce smoke and manage luminal distention.

While not commonly used today, sclerosant injection remains an effective hemostatic therapy. Specifically, absolute ethanol, rather than polidocanol, should be administered. Ethanol sclerotherapy has shown a notable reduction in rebleeding (NNT of 5) and a mortality benefit (NNT of 9), providing strong evidence for its efficacy in treating ulcer bleeding.[88]

Epinephrine injection, on the other hand, should not be used as monotherapy. Studies have shown that epinephrine alone is less effective compared to other monotherapies like thermal contact therapy or clips.[88] Therefore, epinephrine should be combined with another endoscopic hemostatic modality. It's common practice to inject epinephrine before ther-

If epinephrine injection is used, then it should be in combination with another hemostatic modality since epinephrine monotherapy is ineffective

mal contact therapy to reduce bleeding and improve visibility. When combined with clip therapy, it is advisable to inject epinephrine after clip placement to control bleeding if necessary. Injecting epinephrine before clip placement may hinder proper tissue grasping for clip deployment.

Hemostatic powder sprays, such as TC-325, receive a conditional recommendation due to limited data. They can be beneficial for actively bleeding lesions, particularly when other measures fail or for large bleeding areas like actively bleeding neoplasms. As more powder sprays have become available, further trials will help clarify their role in endoscopic hemostasis. However, these sprays are expensive, especially in the United States, so cost considerations are essential.

Over-the-scope clips (OTSCs) function similarly to band ligators by suctioning the bleeding area before deploying a clip. An international multi-center RCT found that OTSCs were superior to through-the-scope clips in reducing rebleeding after initial hemostasis, though there was no significant difference in the need for surgery or mortality.[103] Thus, OTSCs are particularly useful for recurrent ulcer bleeding after initial hemostasis.

In summary, the strongest evidence supports the use of thermal contact therapy and absolute ethanol injection, as recommended by the guidelines. Choose the endoscopic hemostatic therapy you are most comfortable with to maximize the chances of successful hemostasis.

For our patient with the ulcer and its non-bleeding visible vessel, thermal contact therapy was used to effectively seal the vessel. Following this, high-dose PPIs should be administered for 3 days to stabilize the gastric pH and promote clot healing. Numerous trials have shown that PPIs reduce rebleeding, the need for surgery, and mortality more effectively than H2RAs after endoscopic hemostasis. The guidelines strongly rec-ommend high-dose PPI therapy for at least the first 3 days post-hemostasis, either continuous or inter-mittent dosing. A good regimen is 80 mg by bolus on the first day followed by 8 mg/hour infusion or 40 mg 2-4 times per day, intravenously or orally, for the first 3 days. For low-risk stigmata, such as a flat pigmented spot or clean ulcer base, once-daily standard PPI therapy is sufficient. For high-risk endoscopic stigmata, a twice-daily PPI regimen is recommended from days 4 to 14 post-endoscopy to further reduce rebleeding risk, as shown in a prospective RCT from Taiwan.[104] **Figure 3.3** provides a summary of the treatment strategies for each of the 4 major ulcer stigmata.

Figure 3.3. *Endoscopic stigmata and recommended therapy.[81]*

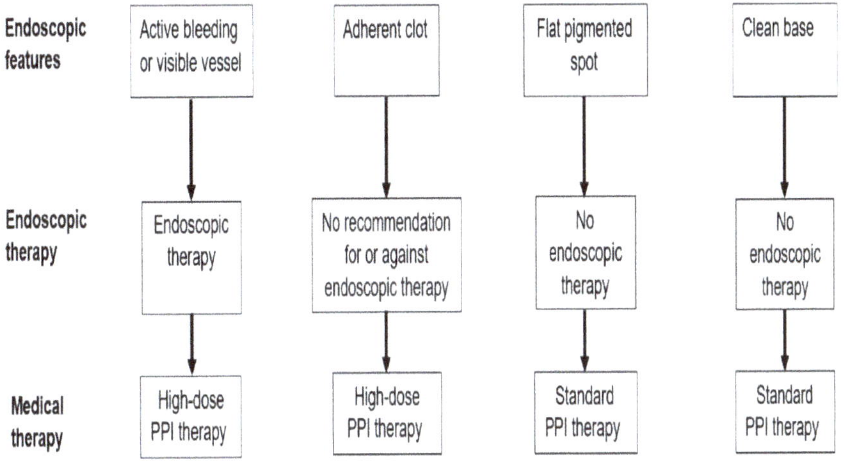

Case 3.4: Upper GI Bleed

You are called by the ED for consultation on a 33-year-old man who has been taking ibuprofen twice daily for the past week after a back injury during snowboarding. He experienced nausea and vomiting with hematemesis, followed by melena last night, which prompted his visit to the ED this morning. Since arriving at the ED, he has not had a bowel movement. He reports no abdominal pain, fever, or lightheadedness.

On examination in the ED, his blood pressure is 112/70 mmHg and heart rate is 88 bpm. His hemoglobin level is 11.2 g/dL. His abdominal examination is unremarkable, and he does not appear ill. He has large-bore IVs placed and is receiving intravenous normal saline.

You perform an EGD later in the afternoon, which shows the following image (**Figure 3.4**) after extensive water jet irrigation.

Know your guidelines!

1. What are you going to do during this EGD?

Figure 3.4. *Peptic ulcer at the pylorus. Image source: J. Andy Tau, MD.*

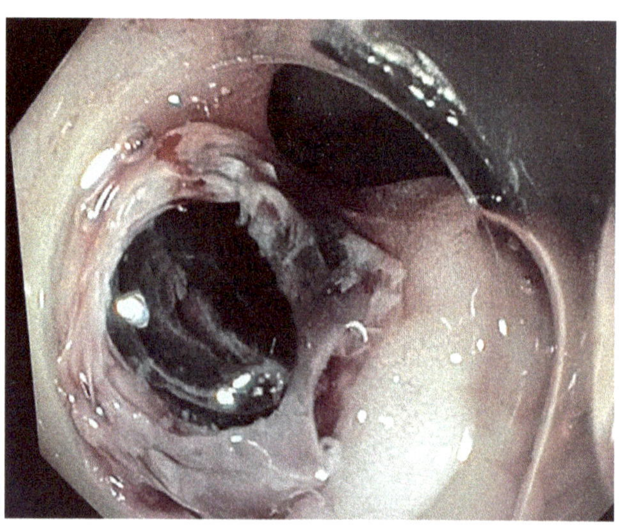

Case 3.4: What do the guidelines say?

Source: ACG 2021 Upper GI and Ulcer Bleeding Guideline[81]

What is that black marble-looking thing in the center of the image? It's important to recognize that this is an adherent clot. But what should be done? Recall that an adherent clot is a Forrest class 2B lesion with approximately a 22% rebleeding risk without endoscopic therapy. Do you take out a cold snare and guillotine it off or just let sleeping dogs lie?

This is where the evidence gets a bit dicey. Studies regarding adherent clots are quite heterogeneous with small sample sizes and differing results, making it difficult to determine which patients may benefit from endoscopic therapy. This uncertainty has led to a standoff in the guidelines. The current expert panel

could not reach a recommendation for or against endoscopic therapy for ulcers with an adherent clot resistant to vigorous irrigation. Previous ACG practice guidelines from 2012 stated that "endoscopic therapy may be considered for patients with an adherent clot resistant to vigorous irrigation,"[105] but the evidence remains inconclusive.

So, what do you do? Again, do what makes you comfortable. It's dealer's choice, and you are the dealer. You hold all the cards. If you want to unroof that clot and see if there's a visible vessel that could be amenable to endoscopic therapy, then go ahead. If you'd rather not deal with endoscopic therapy at this particular point in time, that's fine too. The guidelines give you the flexibility to make the call based on your judgment and comfort level in the given situation.

Case 3.5: Hosing Blood

The last patient with the adherent clot underwent cold snaring and ir-rigation, which revealed a nonbleeding visible vessel. You performed endoscopic hemostasis with a combination of epinephrine injection and heater probe therapy to seal the vessel shut (check out **Figure 3.5**—you can still see some residual smoke after electrocautery). The patient is also on continuous intravenous PPI infusion at 8 mg/hr. Unfortunately, you get the dreaded 2 AM phone call from the ICU: this patient is now "hosing blood" with large volume hematemesis and hematochezia, and the hemoglobin has dropped to 9.1 g/dL (down from 11.2 g/dL prior). Yikes.

Figure 3.5. *Adherent clot before (left image) and after (right image) hemostasis.*
Image source: J. Andy Tau, MD.

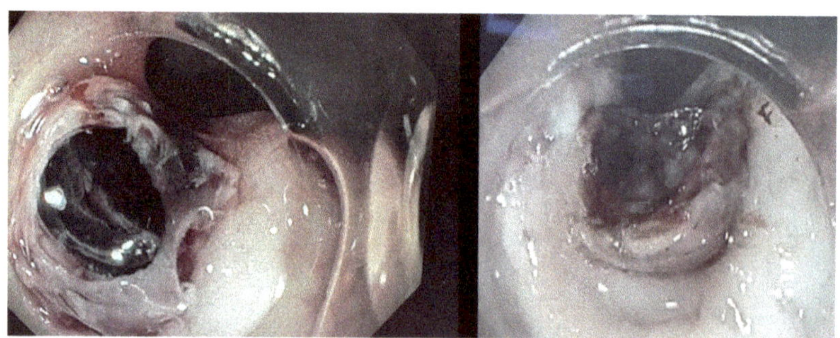

Know your guidelines!

1.   What is your next step?

2.

Case 3.5: What do the guidelines say?

Source: ACG 2021 Upper GI and Ulcer Bleeding Guideline[81]

Even though we're tempted to immediately call interventional radiology (IR) or surgery for help, it's often better to perform a repeat EGD to control the bleeding. A prospective RCT compared repeat EGD with surgery in patients who developed recurrent bleeding after initial endoscopic hemostasis.[106] The trial found that 73% of patients undergoing immediate endoscopic retreatment had effective control of bleeding after the repeat endoscopy with fewer complications compared to the surgery group. However, there were two cases of perforation in the repeat endoscopy group, likely due to repeat thermocoagulation, which then required surgery.

As noted in the guideline, it's worthwhile to use a different form of endoscopic hemostasis (e.g., clips like OTSCs) on a repeat EGD after initial thermocoagulation. Important risk factors for failure of successful repeat endoscopic hemostasis included initial hypotension at the time of rebleeding and ulcer size ≥ 2 cm. So, if you're called about a re-bleeder after successful endoscopic hemostasis, it's crucial to consider if the patient was suddenly hypotensive and had a large ulcer, as this might predict an unsuccessful repeat EGD. It might be prudent to have IR and/or surgery on standby.

Given these findings, the guideline panel recommends that patients with recurrent bleeding after endoscopic therapy for a bleeding ulcer undergo repeat endoscopic therapy rather than surgery or transcatheter arterial embolization (TAE).

What if you can't control the bleeding endoscopically? Instead of running and hiding, the first call should generally be to IR to consider TAE. Historically, we'd call the surgeons for rescue in such cases. However, recent data suggest that IR should try first after endoscopic failure. A meta-analysis[107] and Swedish population-based cohort study[108] showed decreased complications in patients under-going TAE compared to surgery, without an increase in mortality.

Though surgery did show decreased further bleeding compared to TAE, the choice of strategy after endoscopic failure may depend on local expertise and practice patterns. Generally, we should rely on our IR colleagues first before calling in the surgery team. This consensus was supported by the guideline panel, which recommended TAE for bleeding ulcer patients who have failed endoscopic therapy.

Case 3.6: Coagulopathy

A 71-year-old man with a history of atrial fibrillation and aortic aneurysm, on warfarin, presents to the ED with melena and generalized fatigue for the past three days. He has been taking levofloxacin for rhinosinusitis over the past week, which has improved his congestion and drainage. Labs from his primary care physican's office 7 days ago showed:

WBC 11.2, Hgb 14.2, Platelets 181K, INR 2.1, creatinine 1.2.

In the ED, his BP is 78/51, HR 120, and he appears unwell with pallor. His abdomen is soft and not tender or distended. Melenic stool is noted in his rectal vault.

Current labs in the ED reveal:

WBC 10.3, Hgb 9.0, Platelets 194K, INR 4.7.

While in the ED, he immediately receives intravenous fluid boluses, starts on vasopressors, and is admitted to the ICU. You are consulted with a request for an immediate EGD.

Know your guidelines!

1.   Will you be doing the EGD immediately as requested?

2.   How are you going to manage the INR?

3.   What is the next most appropriate step?

Case 3.6: What do the guidelines say?

Source: ACG 2022 Management of Patients on Anticoagulants and Antiplatelets During Acute Gastrointestinal Bleeding and the Peri-Endoscopic Period Guideline[109]

Of course, we want the patient stabilized and adequately resuscitated before performing an EGD. We can tell the ICU team to hold off on the EGD and point to evidence showing that outcomes don't improve with very early endoscopy.[99] We covered this in the ulcer bleeding section earlier, so if you need a refresher, go back and review that vignette. Suffice it to say, the patient will fare better when adequately resuscitated prior to EGD.

Beyond resuscitation, we should address the patient's elevated INR. Ever wonder where warfarin came from? Interestingly, its origins are rooted in Wisconsin agriculture. Moldly hay was causing cows to hemorrhage to death because their blood wouldn't clot. The substance found use as a pesticide, causing rodents to internally hemorrhage, and soon after, it was adopted as a vitamin K antagonist (VKA) for humans. The chemical was named after the Wisconsin Alumni Research Foundation (WARF), which supported its investors. They combined the first 4 letters with the last 2 syllables of coumarin, creating "warfarin." Isn't this book already worth its price just for learning these facts? Anyway...

Quinolones, including levofloxacin, have numerous side effects that are often overlooked. One significant interaction is with warfarin, affecting the cytochrome P450 system. Quinolones inhibit cytochrome P450, displacing warfarin from binding sites and preventing its metabolism, which increases warfarin levels in the bloodstream, leading to a su-pratherapeutic INR.[110,111] Additionally, quinolones are associated with aortic aneurysms and dissection, particularly with levofloxacin. Given this patient's history of an aortic aneurysm on warfarin, levofloxacin was a doubly poor choice. Quinolones also prolong the QT interval, cause tendon rupture (especially the Achilles), increase the risk of *C. difficile* infec-tion, and can lead to peripheral neuropathy. Resistance to quinolones has been rising due to their widespread use, making them less innocuous than once thought.

Returning to our patient, we must first determine if he has life-threatening hemorrhage, defined as major clinically overt bleeding resulting in hypovolemic shock or severe hypotension requiring pressors or surgery, or requiring a transfusion of ≥ 5 units of packed red blood cells, or associated with a decrease in hemoglobin > 5 g/dL, or causing death.[112] A simple way to remember this is the "Rule of Fives," coined by Dr. Neena Abraham, an expert in "cardiogastroenterology" (see **Table 3.5**).

Table 3.5. *"Rule of Fives" criteria to determine if GI bleeding is life-threatening.*

Rule of Fives
Any of the following qualifies to be life-threatening
Decrease in hgb > 5 g/dL
Requirement of ≥ 5 units of packed red blood cells
Hypovolemic shock or requirement for pressors
At risk for causing death

So, this patient qualifies for life-threatening hemorrhage by having a drop in hemoglobin of more than 5 g/dL and requiring pressors, and certainly being at risk for causing death. With that in mind, we need to decide whether VKA (warfarin) reversal is necessary to correct the coagulopathy. The guidelines, reviewed by multiple GRADE (Grad-ing of Recommendations, Assessment, Development, and Evalua-tions) methodologists, provide evidence-based recommendations on the best course of action.

For this patient, vitamin K is not recommended due to its delayed onset of action without significant benefit in the acute setting. It takes a day or 2 for vitamin K to work, and by then, it might be too late. Fresh

Do not give vitamin K or FFP for acute GI bleeding and supra-therapeutic INR frozen plasma (FFP) is also not recommended due to the lack of benefit and potential complications, such as infection transmission, pulmonary edema, and congestive heart failure from the increased volume needed for transfusion. Additionally, FFP carries an increased risk for thrombosis.[113] Back in the day, the knee-jerk response would be to immediately get some FFP thawed out for transfusion. Not anymore.

If FFP isn't the answer, what is the best way to quickly lower the INR? And is it necessary? Most GI bleeds do not require INR correction. However, in a life-threatening GI bleed like this one, INR reversal should certainly be considered. Prothrombin complex concentrate (PCC) tends to be more reliable and rapid with a smaller volume compared to FFP and can be lifesaving, especially useful before endoscopy. If the bleeding is not life-threatening, you can probably hold off on the PCC (there's not enough data for the guideline experts to provide a recommendation for that scenario), but you should definitely not be giving vitamin K or FFP.

It seems like almost every patient admitted to our hospital for a GI bleed is taking a direct oral anticoagulant (DOAC). These are the new generation of non-vitamin K anticoagulants which target a specific factor in the coagulation cascade. These agents (see **Table 3.6**) have a shorter half-life than warfarin, with fewer side effects, including less bleeding and less influence by diet and other medications. They also do not require frequent blood monitoring, so dosing is typically stable. Moreover, they reach therapeutic levels within a few hours rather than days, which means they usually wear off within 1-2 days after the last dose. The currently available DOACs include factor Xa inhibitors (apixaban, rivaroxaban, edoxaban) and one thrombin (factor IIa) inhibitor (dabigatran). A quick way to determine which factor a particular DOAC is inhibiting is to look at the name. The Xa inhibitors have "xa" within their names (e.g., api**xa**ban, rivaro**xa**ban, edo**xa**ban). Factor IIa inhibitors do not.

Table 3.6. *Direct oral anticoagulants (DOACs) and corresponding reversal agent.*

Xa Inhibitors (reversal with andexanet alfa)	IIa Inhibitor (reversal with idarucizumab)
Api**xa**ban	Dabigatran
Rivoro**xa**ban	
Edo**xa**ban	

Notably, all of these DOACs have some renal excretion, meaning they will linger longer in the bloodstream of patients with renal impairment. So, let's say our patient was taking a DOAC instead of warfarin with the same level of life-threatening bleeding. You can opt for a specific reversal agent: andexanet alfa for those on Xa inhibitors and idarucizumab for those on the thrombin inhibitor, dabigatran. These reversal agents are effective but quite expensive and often not readily available due to their infrequent use. If you can't get these agents, PCC can be used as it contains the factors (X and II) inhibited by the DOAC. The guideline panel also suggests this strategy based on available evidence.

What if your patient is experiencing slow or minor bleeding and is not in a life-threatening situation? In this case, if they are on a DOAC, it's best to let the drug wear off naturally without using a specific reversal agent or PCC.

Now, let's consider a patient not severely bleeding but on a VKA like warfarin. In this scenario, you should avoid giving FFP or vitamin K. There isn't enough evidence to recommend PCC for such patients. Guidelines, based on the GRADE methodology, require a solid evidence base to make recommendations, and if the data isn't there, a recommendation can't be made. In this case, simply holding the VKA or warfarin and allowing the INR to decrease naturally is advisable. Time often works well in these situations. To summarize the guideline recommendations, **Figure 3.6** provides a

DOACs will have longer half lives in patients with renal insufficiency

If patient on DOAC is not having life-threatening hemorrhage, then allow spontaneous clearance and do not provide PCC or a specific reversal agent

management algorithm for patients on anticoagulants with acute GI bleeding.

Figure 3.6. *Anticoagulant GI bleeding management algorithm.*[114]

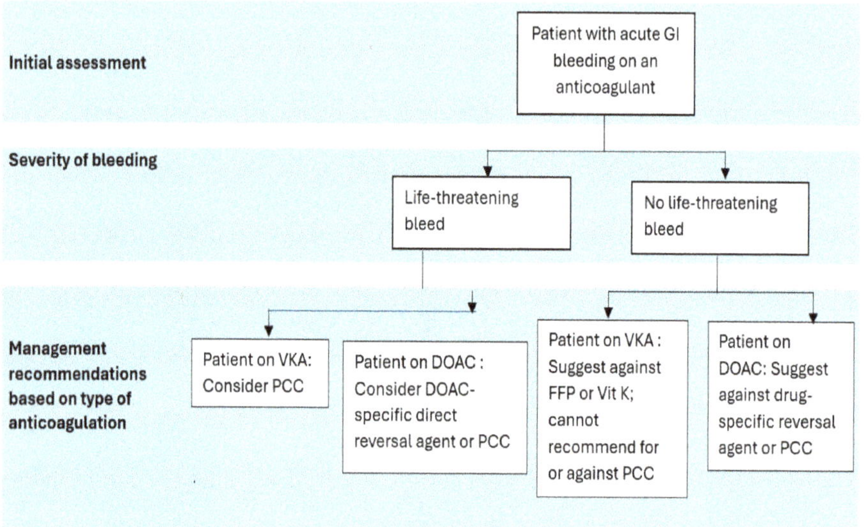

Case 3.7: Platelet Perplexity

A 67-year-old woman with a history of hyperlipidemia and acute coronary syndrome 2 years ago, resulting in coronary stent placement in her left anterior descending artery, has been asymptomatic from a cardiac standpoint since then. She is currently taking aspirin 81 mg, clopidogrel 75 mg, and atorvastatin 40 mg daily. However, she now presents to the ED with acute onset of hematemesis, lightheadedness, and mahogany-colored stools for the past 24 hours. She is ill-appearing with BP 82/29, HR 118. Her abdomen is soft and mildly tender in the epigastrium without rebound or guarding.

Labs: WBC 8.1, Hgb 9.3, platelets 153K, ALT 18, total bilirubin 0.7, Alb 4.2, Cr 0.9, BUN 28, INR 1.0.

CT scan: Normal GI tract, normal liver and spleen, no contrast extravasation, no extraluminal air, no acute abnormalities.

You have advised that once the patient is stabilized, you are planning to perform an EGD. The ED attending has started intravenous flu-ids for resuscitation and intravenous PPI therapy. She has also sent a type and screen for possible future blood transfu-sion. She wants to know if you would like the patient to have a platelet transfusion since she is on dual antiplatelet therapy.

Know your guidelines!

1. Should you start a platelet transfusion?

2. How are you going to manage the dual antiplatelet therapy in the peri-endoscopic period?

Case 3.7: What do the guidelines say?

Source: ACG 2022 Management of Patients on Anticoagulants and Antiplatelets During Acute Gastrointestinal Bleeding and the Peri-Endoscopic Period Guideline[109]

Patients with coronary stents are often placed on dual antiplatelet therapy (DAPT) for secondary prevention of another cardiovascular event. DAPT typically includes acetylsalicylic acid (ASA) in combination with a $P2Y_{12}$ inhibitor, which blocks the specific platelet surface receptor. Clopidogrel and prasugrel are thienopyridine $P2Y_{12}$ inhibitors with an irreversible effect lasting the lifetime of the platelet (about 7 to 10 days). In contrast, ticagrelor is a nonthienopyridine P2Y12 inhibitor with a reversible effect on platelet function, lasting about 3 to 5 days (see **Table 3.7**). Despite these differences, they are quite similar in clinical practice.

Table 3.7. *P2Y12 platelet inhibitors.*

Common P2Y12 inhibitors
Clopidgrel – thienopyridine; irreversible effect
Prasugrel   – thienopyridine; irreversible effect
Ticagrelor – nonthienopyridine; reversible effect

For the cardiovascular protective effects of ASA, 81 mg daily is sufficient, which is why you don't see many people on 325 mg any longer. This discussion is about secondary prophylaxis. Primary prophylaxis of a cardiovascular event with ASA is a different topic, but in brief, it's limited to select populations due to the higher risks of bleeding outweighing cardiovascular benefits for most people.

ASA works by irreversibly inactivating COX-1-dependent thromboxane A2 production, which reduces thromboxane A2's prothrombotic properties like platelet aggregation. Platelets don't express the COX-2 enzyme, which is why COX-2 selective NSAIDs don't affect platelet function and may be linked to increased cardiovascular risks. The irreversible effects on platelets last about a week, corresponding to the platelet lifespan.

High-risk patients for recurrent thrombosis include those with an acute coronary syndrome who had a drug-eluting stent (DES) placed within the past year or a bare-metal stent (BMS) within the past 2 months. [115] Our patient, 2 years post-DES placement, isn't in the highest risk category, but her provider has kept her on DAPT, which is a somewhat common occurrence for ED bleeders.

So, if this patient on antiplatelet medications is actively bleeding without thrombocytopenia, will providing platelet transfusion help? Nope. Platelet transfusion can actually do more harm than good here. A study found that platelet transfusion in this scenario significantly increased mortality (odds ratio 5.6) compared to no transfusion, with a trend towards increased bleeding and thrombosis.[116] Therefore, unless the patient has marked thrombocytopenia with active bleeding, platelet transfusion should be avoided.

What about her DAPT? Should either or both agents be held during active bleed-ing? It makes sense to hold the $P2Y_{12}$ inhibitor (clopidogrel) since she is past the high-risk window for DES placement after acute cor-onary syndrome. However, the guidelines specifically state that ASA should be continued in the face of acute GI bleeding. If stopped, the guidelines recommend resuming ASA on the day endoscopic hemo-stasis is achieved. **Figure 3.7** provides a management algorithm sum-marizing this approach.

Why immediately resume ASA? Recall that the lifespan of a platelet is about a week, and both ASA and clopidogrel are irreversible inhibitors, meaning their effects persist for the duration of the platelet's life. This means that even if these medications are stopped, platelet inhibition will continue for several days. Resuming ASA is crucial for long-term car-diovascular protection.

Evidence supports this approach. In a RCT from Hong Kong, a well-known center for GI bleeding re-search, 156 patients on 80 mg of ASA daily for secondary prophylaxis were treated with

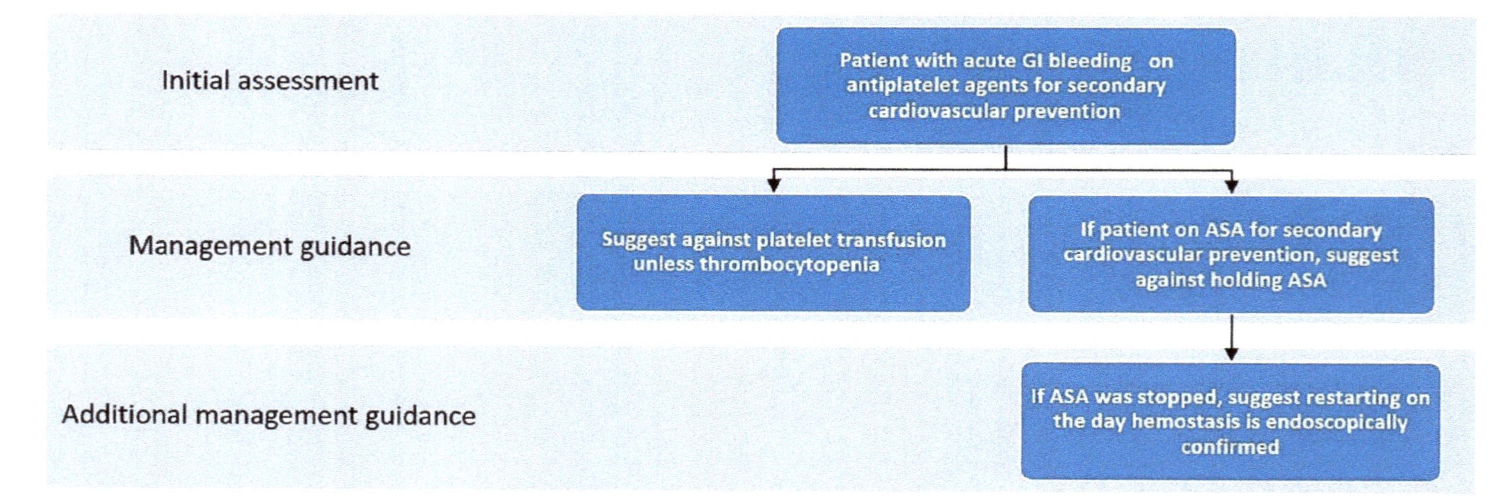

Figure 3.7. *Antiplatelet GI bleeding treatment algorithm.*[114]

endoscopic hemostasis and PPI.117 They were then randomized to continue low-dose ASA or placebo for 8 weeks immediately after hemostasis. Although the 30-day recurrent bleed-ing rate was numerically higher in the ASA group, it was not sta-tistically significant. However, the all-cause mortality rate attributed to cardiovascular, cerebrovascular, or gastrointestinal complications was significantly lower in the ASA group (1.3%) compared to the placebo group (10.3%) (**Figure 3.8**). Thus, resuming ASA as soon as hemostasis is confirmed in the setting of acute GI bleeding is essential. It's much easier and better to manage GI bleeding than to deal with potentially devastating cardiovascular thromboses. After all, the heart is more important than the gut!

Figure 3.8. *Insignificant 30-day rebleeding, but significant mortality reduction in aspirin group vs placebo after endoscopic hemostasis.*[117]

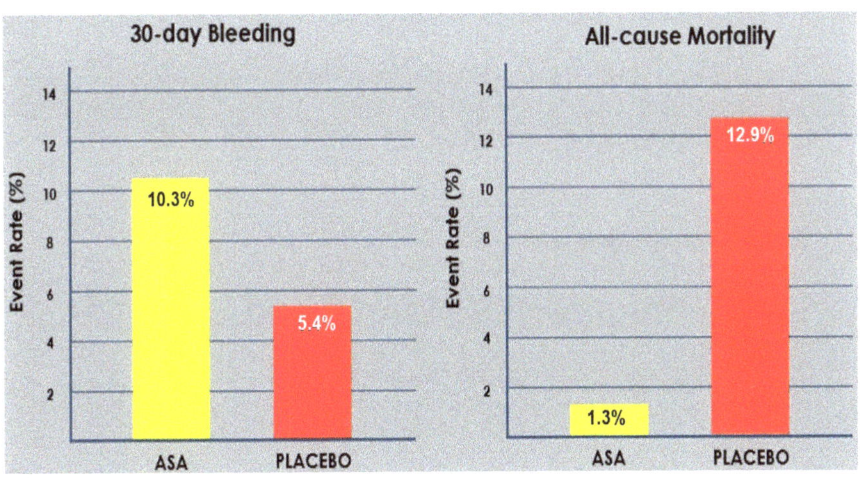

Case 3.8: March Madness

A 62-year-old woman with a history of myocardial infarction and DES placement in her left main coronary artery on New Year's Day has been on ASA 81 mg daily and ticagrelor 90 mg twice daily. Since 2 months have passed and it is now March—colon cancer awareness month—she is particularly concerned about colon cancer. She recalls that you removed adenomatous colon polyps during her colonoscopy 7 years ago, and her mother had colon cancer at age 56. She would like to have a colonoscopy now.

She has no change in bowel habits, rectal bleeding, anemia, abdominal pain, or weight loss. She mentions that she has felt great since her cardiac intervention and has remained asymptomatic. She exercises routinely, including jogging three miles every other day without chest pain, lightheadedness, or palpitations. In the office today, she looks very well, with unremarkable vital signs and normal laboratory tests. She also explains that she is changing jobs this month, with her future health insurance being uncertain, and terms it "March Madness." Therefore, she really wants to get her colonoscopy done within the next couple of weeks.

Know your guidelines!

1. Should you proceed with colonoscopy now?

2. What is the next most appropriate step?

Case 3.8: What do the guidelines say?

Source: ACG 2022 Management of Patients on Anticoagulants and Antiplatelets During Acute Gastrointestinal Bleeding and the Peri-Endoscopic Period Guideline[109]

It might be good to think of the motto "all good things come to those who wait" for this case. If you recall, this patient is at high risk for a recurrent thrombotic cardiovascular event due to having a DES placed recently after an ACS. That's why she is on DAPT with ASA in combination with a $P2Y_{12}$ inhibitor. Those with DES are at higher risk of thrombosis compared to those with a bare-metal stent (BMS). If this pa-tient had a BMS, then it would be advised to defer elective procedures for 2 months with ACS and 1 month without ACS. Since she had a DES placed in conjunction with ACS (myocardial infarction), elective procedures should be deferred for 12 months—6 months for those with with DES without ACS.[111]

Stay tuned for updates as these time intervals may shorten in future guidelines, with studies proposing that monotherapy with a $P2Y_{12}$ platelet inhibitor conversion from DAPT within 3 months af-ter DES placement for ACS may suffice.[118,119] At any rate, it would be wise at this point to wait for one year after the initial DES place-ment in this case. Even though she feels great and looks well, she is at high risk for thrombus without DAPT so soon after ACS and DES placement. Thus, deferment is the best option here as this is truly an elective procedure. She certainly has an increased risk of developing colon cancer (check out *G2G Volume 1* for more on that), but the colonoscopy can wait. Her insurance status should not play a role in determining the proper timeframe for performing an elective proce-dure in a safe manner.

Let's assume that the proper time interval has passed, and it is now acceptable to proceed with colonoscopy. How are you going to manage her DAPT in the periprocedural window? First and foremost, you need input from her cardiologist or hematologist before scheduling the procedure. Typically, you would then make a shared decision to hold the P2Y$_{12}$ inhibitor for up to a week and continue the baby ASA throughout the periprocedural time (**Figure 3.9**). However, if there is concern for postprocedural bleeding such as a high-risk procedure (e.g., large endoscopic mucosal resection), the guidelines do provide some wiggle room to make a case-by-case determination on when to resume the P2Y$_{12}$ inhibitor. Perhaps you may want to hold the P2Y$_{12}$ inhibitor for a few days or even a week.

Figure 3.9. *Dual antiplatelet therapy (DAPT) management for elec-tive endoscopy.*[114]

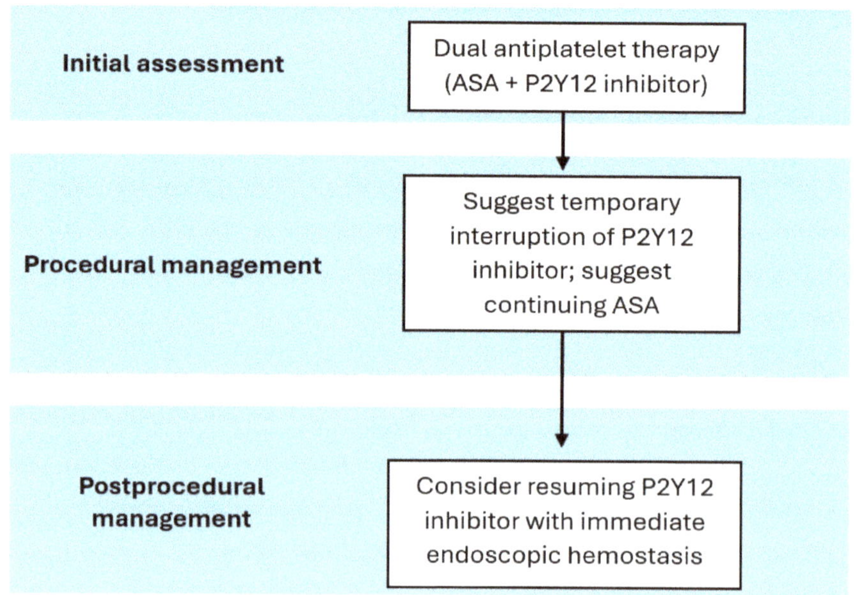

Case 3.9: PEG Placement

A 67-year-old man with a history of chronic atrial fibrillation and a cerebrovascular accident (CVA) 6 months ago presents with progressive dysphagia and difficulty initiating swallows. Despite speech and swallow therapy, his symptoms have minimally improved. Over the past 2 months, he has experienced significant weight loss of 13 lbs due to insufficient caloric intake. You are consulted to consider an EGD and percutaneous endoscopic gastrostomy (PEG) tube placement.

His past surgical history includes a laparoscopic appendectomy and open left inguinal hernia repair. He has no history of hypertension, diabetes, congestive heart failure, renal insufficiency, coronary artery disease, or peripheral arterial disease. He is currently taking rivaroxaban 20 mg every evening. On examination, he is afebrile with an irregularly irregular pulse at 80 bpm and a blood pressure of 127/73 mmHg. His oxygen saturation is 99% on room air. His abdomen is soft and non-tender, with well-healed surgical scars from previous operations, but otherwise unremarkable.

Know your guidelines!

1.   Is it appropriate to place a PEG now?

2.   How are you going to manage the anticoagulant?

3.   Is bridging with low molecular weight heparin needed?

Case 3.9: What do the guidelines say?

Source: ACG 2022 Management of Patients on Anticoagulants and Antiplatelets During Acute Gastrointestinal Bleeding and the Peri-Endoscopic Period Guideline[109]

We are often faced with a consult like this, which can be challenging when determining the optimal timing for PEG placement and managing anticoagulation in the periprocedural period. When dealing with patients on anticoagulants or antiplatelet agents, it's crucial to involve cardiology or hematology colleagues for risk stratification and shared decision-making with the patient and their family. This involves understanding both thromboembolic and bleeding risks.

We are not cardiologists or hematologists, but some basic knowledge of thromboembolic risk is crucial. For example, mechanical heart valves (especially mitral) with a history of atrial fibrillation and recent stroke, transient ischemic attack (TIA), or thromboembolism place patients at higher risk. Familiarity with the CHA_2DS_2-VASc risk score for nonvalvular atrial fibrillation is essential, as it helps us understand the patient's stroke risk. The more risk factors a patient has, the higher the thromboembolic risk (see **Table 3.8**). This knowledge helps in balancing the risks and forming a plan for anticoagulation management during the procedure.

Regarding procedural bleeding risk, this is our area of expertise. We need to estimate this part of the equation ourselves, as we are the ones performing the procedures. Balancing these risks allows us to create a safe and effective game plan for managing anticoagulation around the procedure.

Table 3.8. *Positive CHA$_2$DS$_2$-VASc risk factors for thromboembolism in nonvalvular atrial fibrillation.*

CHA$_2$DS$_2$-VASc Score Positive Risk Factors
Congestive heart failure
Hypertension
Age > 64
Diabetes mellitus
Stroke/TIA/thromboembolism
Vascular disease (prior myocardial infarction, arterial disease)
Sex (female)

The endoscopic risk of bleeding varies with the type of procedure being contemplated. Fortunately, the guideline authors and expert consensus provided a list (**Table 3.9**) that stratifies the high versus low/moderate bleeding risks associated with different endoscopic procedures. Keep in mind that as endoscopic techniques improve (e.g., the use of mechanical clips), the bleeding risk should decrease for many of the advanced procedures. Thus, expect changes as time goes by.

Back to our case. Our patient has a moderate thromboembolic risk based on his positive risk factors (age and prior CVA) and faces a high bleeding risk with PEG placement. Before the procedure, you want to ensure that his rivaroxaban is held for a full 1-2 days since he has normal renal function. After successfully placing the PEG, you might want to hold the DOAC for up to 2 additional days, depending on how smoothly the PEG placement went. You don't want to hold the DOAC much more than 2-3 days after the procedure, as this would increase the patient's risk for thrombosis. As you know, DOACs reach peak plasma concentration within a few hours after resuming. Thus, bridging with low molecular weight heparin is not necessary. With a high bleeding risk procedure, you may want that extra time to ensure that there has been adequate

Table 3.9. *Empiric endoscopic procedural bleeding risk stratification.*[109]

High bleeding risk procedures (30-d risk of major bleed > 2%)	Low/moderate bleeding risk procedures (30-d risk of major bleed ≤2%)
Polypectomy (≥ 1cm)	EGD with/without biopsy
PEG/PEJ placement	Colonoscopy with/without biopsy
ERCP with biliary or pancreatic sphincterotomy	Flexible sigmoidoscopy with/without biopsy
EMR/ESD	ERCP with stent (biliary or pancreatic) placement or papillary balloon dilation without sphincterotomy
EUS-FNA	EUS without FNA
Endoscopic hemostasis (excluding APC)	Push enteroscopy and diagnostic balloon-assisted enteroscopy
Radiofrequency ablation	Enteral stent deployment
POEM	Argon plasma coagulation
Treatment of varices (including variceal band ligation)	Balloon dilation of luminal stenoses
Therapeutic balloon-assisted enteroscopy	Polypectomy (<1 cm)
Tumor ablation	ERCP without biliary or pancreatic sphincterotomy
Cystgastrostomy	Marking (including clipping, electrocoagulation, tattooing)
Ampullary resection	Video capsule endoscopy
Pneumatic or bougie dilation	
Laser ablation and coagulation	

The sources used for the empiric classification of procedures included the International Society on Thrombosis and Haemostasis Guidance statement, the BRIDGE trial, previously published guidelines, and expert opinion by the authors. APC, argon plasma coagulation; EGD, esophagogastroduodenoscopy; EMR, endoscopic mucosal resection; ERCP, endoscopic retrograde cholangiopancreatography; ESD, endoscopic submucosal dissection; EUS, endoscopic ultrasound; FNA, fine needle aspirate; PEG, percutaneous endoscopic gastrostomy; PEJ, percutaneous endoscopic jejunostomy; POEM, peroral endoscopic myotomy.

clotting and hemostasis. **Figure 3.10** shows the DOAC algorithm for elective endoscopy.

Figure 3.10. *Direct oral anticoagulant (DOAC) management for elective endoscopy.*[114]

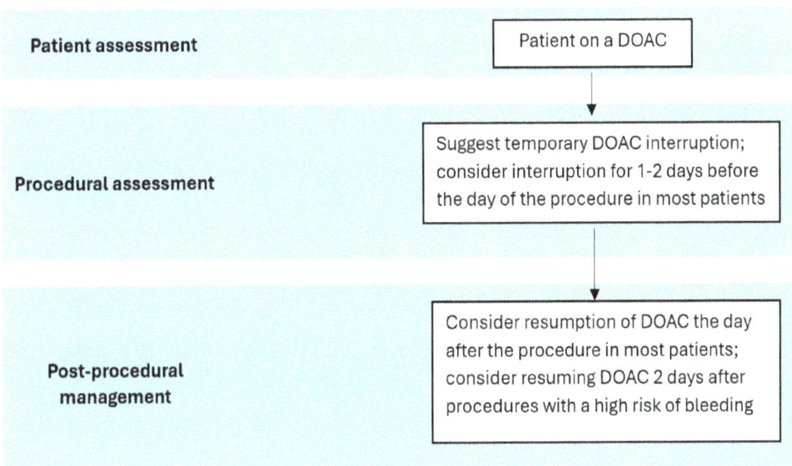

What if the patient was taking warfarin? Given that this is a higher bleeding risk procedure, the guideline panel recommends temporary interruption of the VKA for 5 days prior to the procedure without bridging heparin therapy for most patients. It turns out that bridging with heparin for VKA is not helpful for the vast majority of patients, as noted by two large multi-center RCTs.[120,121] In fact, bridging seems appropriate for only a small subset of patients at the highest risk for thromboembolic events, which is where you need to get input from your cardiology and/or hematology colleagues. Immediately after the procedure, VKA should be resumed, given the long half-life and increased time required to obtain adequate serum anticoagulation.

In summary, don't forget that it is much easier to deal with GI bleeding than it is to correct a CVA, myocardial infarction, or death from a cardiovascular event.

Most patients on VKA do not require heparin bridge prior to elective procedures

Case 3.10: Hematochezia recurrence

A 38-year-old woman with a history of hypertension presents to the ED with painless rectal bleeding, reminiscent of a previous episode from last year. During that incident, she was briefly admitted and underwent a colonoscopy to the terminal ileum, which revealed 2 nonbleeding medium-sized arteriovenous malformations (AVMs) in the ascending colon. There were no diverticula, polyps, or hemorrhoids observed. She was discharged the day after her colonoscopy as her hemoglobin levels remained stable and she did not require a transfusion.

This time, she noted fecal urgency with bright red blood in the commode this morning. Since then, she has not had another bowel movement and immediately presented to the ED, where rectal examination confirmed the presence of blood. She is currently on lisinopril 10 mg daily for hypertension and has recently started ASA 81 mg daily for stroke prevention. She has no family history of cardiovascular disease or colon cancer and reports no fatigue, lightheadedness, or abdominal pain.

On examination, she is afebrile with BP 162/83, HR 86, respiratory rate 12, and 99% oxygen saturation on room air. She appears some-what anxious, and her abdomen is soft and non-tender.

Labs: WBC 7.2, Hemoglobin 13.9, platelets 209, INR 1.0, creatinine 0.8.

Know your guidelines!

1. Do you recommend urgent colonoscopy?

2. Should she be admitted?

3. How do you manage her aspirin therapy?

4. What is the next appropriate step?

Case 3.10: What do the guidelines say?

Source: ACG 2023 Management of patients with acute lower gastrointestinal bleeding: An updated ACG guideline[122]

Believe it or not, it would be safe to send this patient home. Similar to the GBS for upper GI tract bleeding, there's a validated scoring system to prognosticate lower GI bleeding as well. Developed by Kathryn Oakland and colleagues from London, this tool helps determine which patients can be safely discharged for outpatient follow-up and which ones should be admitted.[123]

The Oakland score is straightforward, requiring only simple clinical variables and a hemoglobin value. Add up the designated points, and you get the total score (**Table 3.10**). The key number to remember is an Oakland score of ≤ 8, which equates to a 95% probability of a safe discharge (similar to a GBS of 0 or 1 for upper GI bleeding). A 95% "safe" discharge means there's a 95% chance that the patient won't need readmission within the next 4 weeks for re-bleeding, transfusion, intervention, or death.

Oakland and colleagues also validated this scoring system in the United States with a multicenter study involving over 38,000 patients. They found that an Oakland score ≤ 8 was 98% sensitive for a safe discharge in this population. Extending the score to ≤ 10 yielded a 96% sensitivity for a safe discharge, allowing for the identification of more low-risk patients who don't require hospitalization.

Of course, guidelines are suggestions, not absolutes. Clinical judgment is always the trump card for making the best decisions for individual patients.

This patient doesn't need another colonoscopy since her previous high-quality exam excluded neoplasia and IBD. Her bleeding is likely due to her known AVMs. Discontinue the aspirin used for primary

Table 3.10. *Oakland score variables.*[124]

Variable	Score component value
Age group, y	
≤39	0
40-69	1
≥70	2
Sex	
Female	0
Male	1
Previous hospital admission with LGIB	
No	0
Yes	1
DRE results	
No blood	0
Blood	1
Heart rate, beats/min	
≤69	0
70-89	1
90-109	2
≥110	3
Systolic blood pressure, mm Hg	
50-89	5
90-119	4
120-129	3
130-159	2
≥160	0
Hemoglobin concentration, g/dL	
3.6-6.9	22
7.0-8.9	17
9.0-10.9	13
11.0-12.9	8
13.0-15.9	4
≥16.0	0
DRE, digital rectal examination; LGIB, lower gastrointestinal bleeding	

cardiovascular prophylaxis since it's probably causing her gastrointestinal hemorrhage. If she continues to bleed, a repeat colonoscopy for hemostasis with argon plasma coagulation of the AVMs is warranted. However, if she's on aspirin for secondary prophylaxis, she should continue taking it due to the risk of future cardiovascular thrombosis. A retrospective study from Hong Kong showed that while aspirin use was an independent predictor of rebleeding, it protected against cardiovascular events and death.[125] You can reassure her that she can be discharged and follow up as an outpatient. Plus, you will avoid an unnecessary hospital stay and save healthcare costs.

Case 3.11: Sunday Bloody Sunday

A 79-year-old man with a history of hyperlipidemia, hypertension, and myocardial infarction 5 months ago with a BMS in his left circumflex coronary artery is brought to the ED by his wife after collapsing on the commode following marked painless hematochezia this Sunday afternoon. He mentions that he was listening to his favorite U2 album when he suddenly felt fecal urgency. After going to the bathroom, he felt lightheaded and slumped over but did not lose consciousness. He denies chest pain, shortness of breath, palpitations, fever, nausea, or abdominal pain. His wife immediately drove him to the ED.

On arrival, his vitals are: temperature 36.7°C, BP 87/61, HR 92, RR 14, and 100% oxygen saturation on room air. He appears fatigued but not toxic. His abdomen is soft, nontender, and nondistended.

He has a primary care outpatient visit summary from last week with routine labs: WBC 6.1, Hgb 12.9, platelets 177K, BUN 19, creatinine 1.0. His current medications are listed as clopidogrel 75 mg dai-ly, ASA 81 mg daily, rosuvastatin 20 mg daily, and metoprolol 50 mg twice daily.

Labs today in the ED: WBC 8.9, Hgb 7.4, platelets 183K, BUN 45, creatinine 1.2.

Know your guidelines!

1.   Do you recommend urgent colonoscopy?

2.   How do you manage his antiplatelet therapy?

3.   What are the next appropriate steps?

Case 3.11: What do the guidelines say?

Source: ACG 2023 Management of patients with acute lower gastrointestinal bleeding: An updated ACG guideline.[122]

There's a lot to do and plenty to think about for this case. This patient is experiencing serious, life-threatening bleeding (an acute 5-gram drop in hemoglobin) and things could deteriorate quickly. He is not technically tachycardic, likely due to the beta blockade effect of metoprolol. Immediate volume resuscitation is necessary, and 2 large-bore IVs should be placed right away.

A restrictive red blood cell transfusion policy to 7 g/dL has shown mortality benefit[85], but this patient needs a transfusion now given his history of ischemic coronary artery disease and significant bleeding, despite his hemoglobin being over 7 g/dL. With equilibration after adequate resuscitation, you know that hemoglobin level will only decrease further. Thus, you want to get the hemoglobin over 8 g/dL for this patient. Go back and check out the upper GI bleeding section for a refresher on this topic.

This patient had acute coronary syndrome with a BMS 5 months ago, so he is now about 3 months out of the high-risk window for thrombosis. Therefore, he should not need to be on DAPT in the face of GI bleeding. In fact, the guidelines specifically mention that $P2Y_{12}$ inhibitors, such as clopidogrel, should be held, and ASA continued if possible. Obviously, if there is torrential bleeding, the cardiologist may decide to hold the ASA too! But even if both ASA and clopidogrel are held, the DAPT effect is going to last for about a week. Flip back a few pages as we covered the management of DAPT with GI bleeding earlier.

Just in case you were wondering, there have not been any antifibrinolytic agents that have proven useful for lower GI bleeding. In particular, tranexamic acid has been the most studied with RCTs[126,127]; however, there have not been improvements in bleeding or mortality. In fact, there have been increased thromboembolic events and even seizures noted. Thus, the guidelines recommend against the administration of antifibrinolytic agents in lower GI bleeding.

Diverticular hemorrhage is by far the most common cause of acute lower GI bleeding in adults.[128] It is important to keep that in mind whenever you are faced with this scenario. However, it is also crucial to know that brisk upper GI bleeding, such as an actively bleeding duodenal ulcer, can produce marked hematochezia. He certainly has risk factors for peptic ulcer disease, including DAPT with a significantly elevated BUN. Thus, performing an EGD is a good idea to do once there has been adequate resuscitation and hemodynamic stabilization if possible. This is mentioned in the management algorithm in the guidelines, shown below in **Figure 3.11.**

Figure 3.11. *Severe hematochezia management algorithm.*[122]

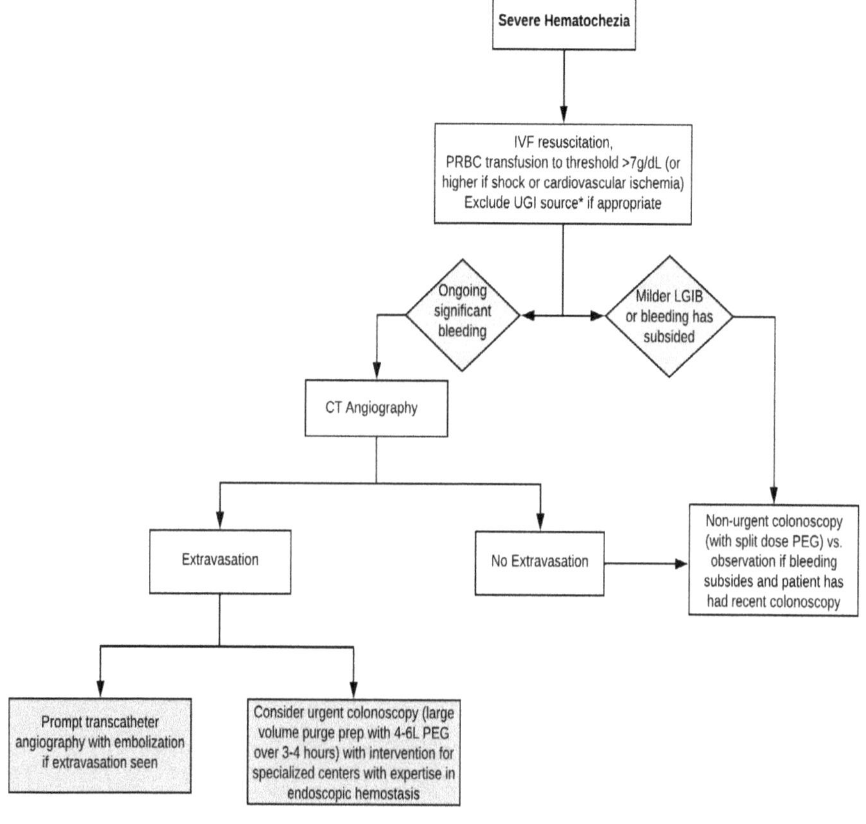

The next step is a computed tomographic angiography (CTA), ideally performed within 4 hours of the last hematochezia to best demonstrate active bleeding via contrast extravasation. This step is crucial as it guides subsequent targeted therapy with prompt transcatheter angiography/arteriography and embolization for hemostasis. Coordinating with IR to ensure they can perform the arteriogram within 90 minutes is essential, as the likelihood of detecting the bleeding site decreases with time.[130] In this case, our IR team successfully embolized a small branch of the inferior mesenteric artery to control the bleeding from a descending colon diverticulum (**Figure 3.12**).

Historically, urgent colonoscopy was the primary method for diagnosing and treating acute lower GI bleeding.[131] However, CTA has largely replaced it due to several advantages. CTA does not require bowel preparation, allowing for a timelier procedure, while urgent colonoscopy necessitates clearing all fecal matter and blood, which is impractical in emergent settings. Achieving hemostasis through urgent colonoscopy is rare; a review of the Clinical Outcomes Research Initiative (CORI) database showed that less than 5% of patients undergoing urgent colonoscopy for severe hematochezia received endoscopic hemostasis.[132] This low success rate underscores the shift towards CTA for initial evaluation and management. If all else fails, surgical intervention remains the last resort.

Figure 3.12. *CT angiogram with subsequent inferior mesenteric angiogram.*[122]

Top Panel: (a) and (b) Coronal CTA images demonstrating contrast accumulation within the left colon.

Bottom Panel: (a) Fluoroscopic inferior mesenteric artery angiogram. (b) Angiogram image obtained several seconds later shows contrast accumulation within the lumen of the descending colon (arrow). (c) Fluoroscopic image obtained showing embolization coils (arrows) within the artery supplying the bleeding diverticulum.

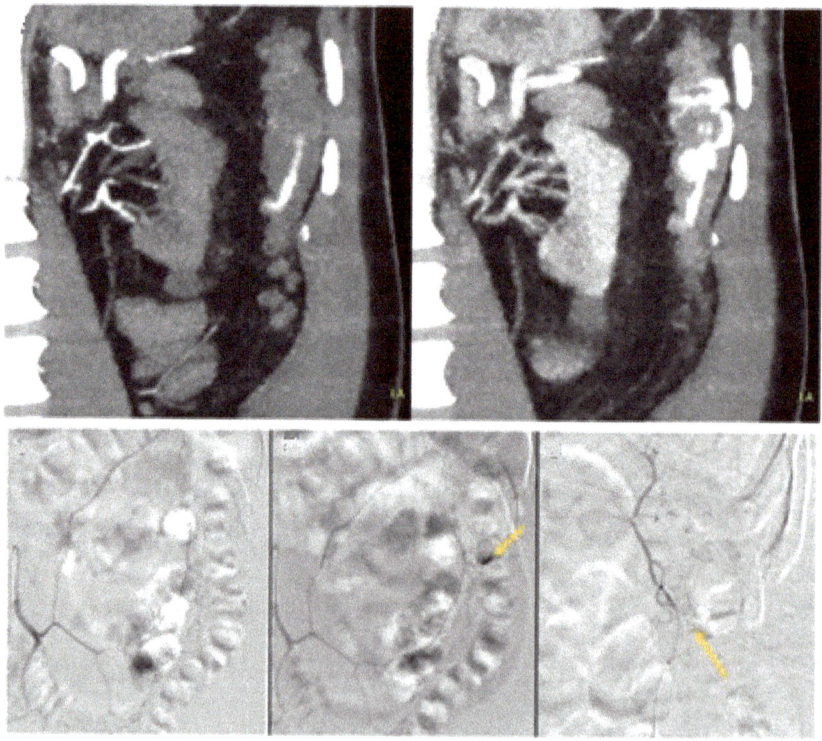

Case 3.12: Tic-Tac-Toe

A 69-year-old woman presents to the ED with hematochezia, which began abruptly the day after she accidentally stepped on a tack 3 days ago. She reported brisk bleeding that came and went in waves over the past 2 days. She has been taking naproxen twice daily for toe pain. Currently, she feels fatigued and lightheaded upon standing, though she has not been standing much due to her toe pain. She has no abdominal pain, rectal pain, tenesmus, or fever. She has a history of diverticulosis noted on a colonoscopy 7 years ago, without hemorrhoids. Her medical history includes chronic atrial fibrillation, for which she takes warfarin daily.

In the ED, her vitals are: Temperature 37.0°C, BP 108/71, HR 102, RR 13, with 98% oxygen saturation on room air. She appears ill, with a soft, non-tender, non-distended abdomen. Rectal exam is deferred as she shows you a large amount of red clots in the bedside commode.

Labs in the ED: WBC 6.4, Hgb 9.7, platelets 212K, BUN 14, creatinine 1.1, INR 2.4, total bilirubin 0.8, albumin 4.1, ALT 19, AST 21.

A stat CT angiogram shows no extravasation of contrast but reveals stool in the colon and diverticular disease without mural thickening. She is admitted to the hospital ward on a clear liquid diet and re-ceives volume resuscitation.

Repeat labs: Hgb 8.6 g/dL, INR 2.3.

Later that evening, the hospital nurse calls you because the patient has passed another large volume bloody bowel movement. He wants to know what you would like to do next.

Know your guidelines!

1.   Does the INR need correction?

2.   Should you observe?

3.   What are your next steps?

Case 3.12: What do the guidelines say?

Source: ACG 2023 Management of patients with acute lower gastrointestinal bleeding: An updated ACG guideline.[122]

Here we have another complicated case with a lot going on and a cloudy picture. However, applying the evidence-based guidelines can clear things up nicely. Firstly, she should stop taking naproxen as it is not cardioprotective and may have precipitated the bleeding. Instead, she can take acetaminophen as needed for her toe pain. Given her recurrent bleeding, she should have an inpatient colonoscopy, but this doesn't need to be done urgently. Recent studies, including a meta-analysis and systematic review,[133] have shown that early or urgent colonoscopy within 24 hours does not improve clinical outcomes such as further bleeding or mortality in hospitalized patients with acute lower GI bleeding. This shift in the paradigm allows for ensuring the patient is hemodynamically optimized and has a well-cleansed bowel, ideally with a split-dose regimen for better results and fewer side effects.

Regarding her elevated INR of 2.3 from warfarin use, it doesn't need to be reversed since endoscopic hemostasis is considered safe and effective with an INR ≤ 2.5. Attempting to normalize the INR could delay endoscopy and potential hemostasis without reducing the rebleeding risk. However, if her INR were supratherapeutic, 4-factor prothrombin complex concentrate (PCC) would be preferred over fresh frozen plasma due to its quicker action and fewer side effects.

For the colonoscopy, use a clear cap on the tip of the colonoscope to help identify and treat the bleeding site, likely a diverticular bleed. Be prepared for hemostasis if you encounter stigmata of recent hemorrhage[128] (**Figure 3.13**).

218

Figure 3.13. *Stigmata of recent diverticular hemorrhage.*[128]
(a) Active arterial bleeding from the diverticular base. (b) Nonbleeding visible vessel at the diverticular neck. (c) Adherent clot in the diverticular base. (d) Flat spot in the diverticular base.

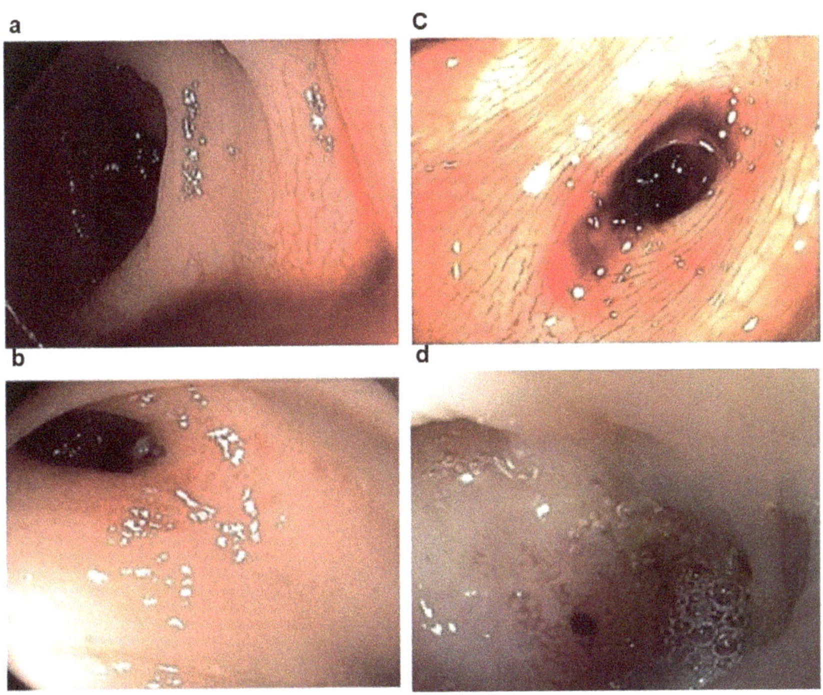

Endoscopic therapy is effective for treating diverticular bleeding stigmata, including bipolar coagulation, clips, and endoscopic band ligation (EBL). It's important to remember that the base of a diverticulum lacks a muscular wall, so a contact thermal coagulation probe should only be applied to the neck of a bleeding diverticulum and not the base. If bleeding stigmata are observed at the base, clips or EBL should be used, with a preference for direct placement over the vessel (**Figure 3.14**).[134] Clips are beneficial for marking the bleeding site, aiding in localization if angiography is needed for rebleeding. Recent data indicates that EBL

> Bipolar coagulation is used for a vessel on the neck of a bleeding diverticulum (not the base)

is not only effective but may be the preferred strategy for reducing diverticular rebleeding. [134,135]

Figure 3.14. *Endoscopic diverticulum band ligation.*[130]

(a) Placement of marking clip lateral to the bleeding diverticulum. (b) EBL device attached to the tip of the scope. (c) EBL completed which involved the bleeding point at the base of the diverticulum.

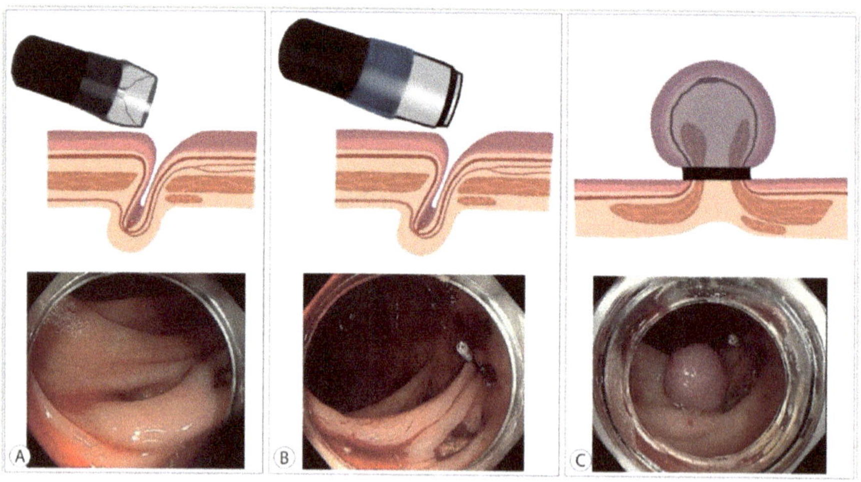

Case 3.13: The Crimson Colon

A 76-year-old woman presents to the ED with sudden onset left lower quadrant abdominal pain, cramping, and several episodes of loose, bloody stools over the past 24 hours. She has a history of hypertension, diabetes, and coronary artery disease, for which she takes aspirin and a beta-blocker. She does not report any recent travel, antibiotic use, or changes in diet.

On physical exam, she's afebrile but appears uncomfortable. Her abdomen is tender to palpation, particularly in the left lower quadrant, with mild guarding but no rebound tenderness. Labs reveal a mild leukocytosis, elevated lactate, and normal liver tests. Her hemoglobin and serum creatinine are within normal limits.

Know your guidelines!

1. What test is indicated now?

2. What might that test reveal

Case 3.13: What do the guidelines say?

Source: ACG 2015 Colon Ischemia guidelines [137]

This patient needs a CT scan. Why? Because there are several features of this story concerning for colon ischemia (CI). This patient has lower abdominal pain and rectal bleeding in the setting of cardiovascular risk factors (hypertension, atherosclerosis, diabetes) and older age. That should make you think of an ischemic origin for both the pain and the bleeding. Of note, the ACG guidelines (and the authors of this book) prefer the term CI over the more commonly used term "ischemic colitis," as the latter connotes ulceration and inflammation. In fact, many people with CI do not yet have a clear inflammatory process when first diagnosed, and instead simply have a reduction in adequate blood flow, leading to ischemic changes. "Colopathy" is a related term that does not imply inflammatory changes and simply refers to subepithelial hemorrhage or edema in the colon. In any event, we want to make this clear distinction because we happen to know that the first author of the ACG CI guidelines, the legendary Larry Brandt, is an expert etymologist and would want to ensure we get it right!

CI arises from changes in systemic circulation or mesenteric vasculature, leading to local hypoperfusion and reperfusion injury. Often, no specific cause is found, suggesting small-vessel disease and nonocclusive ischemia, a form of ischemia the ACG guidelines call "Type I" CI. In contrast, so-called "Type II" CI is linked to systemic hypotension, reduced cardiac output, or aortic surgery. While this classification isn't widely used clinically, it guides treatment approaches, as we'll discuss below.

The disease typically is segmental, which is very important clinically. Although the left colon is most commonly involved, as seems the case in this vignette, all parts of the colon can be affected. CI isolated to the right colon, also called "IRCI," is especially concerning because it is associated with higher mortality when compared to other segments. Clinically, IRCI patients tend to have more abdominal pain and less rectal bleeding than individuals with left-sided colitis, again suggesting that the current case is unlikely to be IRCI. These patients also tend to have more severe cardiovascular disease, atrial fibrillation, and renal disease than those with other forms of CI.[139] When the right colon is involved, it can act more like acute mesenteric ischemia, a related condition in which the superior mesenteric artery and its branches are acutely obstructed, often by an embolus. Although IRCI is different from mesenteric infarction, both have a much more severe disease course than typical CI, which is usually transient and non-fatal (although not always).

While we're on the topic of CI across colon segments, the watershed areas, including the splenic flexure (also called "Griffith's point") and the sigmoid colon (called "Sudeck's point" for all you ACG Jeopardy scholars), are at high risk for mesenteric hypoperfusion. In contrast, the rectum is not typically affected by CI because of its dual blood supply. Finally, when the entire colon is involved (i.e., "pancolonic CI"), which occurs rarely, the outcome can also be very severe, on par with IRCI outcomes.

Risk factors for CI include advanced age, cardiovascular diseases like hypertension and atherosclerosis, diabetes, and a history of bowel surgery. Conditions causing systemic hypotension, such as heart failure or severe dehydration, also elevate the risk. A wide range of medications has also been linked to CI, with varying levels of supporting evidence. This guideline emphasizes that constipation-inducing drugs, immunomodulatory drugs, and illicit drugs like amphetamines and cocaine are most likely to be etiologic, rather than merely associated. **Figure 3.15** provides a mnemonic to learn the medications associated with CI.

Additionally, hypercoagulable states, prolonged physical exertion (e.g., marathon running), and atrial fibrillation, can contribute to the development of CI. Epidemiologically, there is also an interesting link between IBS and CI. It's unclear exactly why IBS might be a risk factor, but it's possible that constipation, with or without fecal impaction, contributes to a heightened risk of CI by elevating intra-colonic pressure and thereby diminishing blood flow due to fecal impaction. This is speculative on our part, but it might also relate to abnormalities in serotonin regulation, a neurotransmitter affecting vascular tone that is known to be dysregulated in IBS. Not sure. In any event, here's that list of medications associated with CI.

Figure 3.15. *Memory aid for medications associated with CI. It spells out COLON ISCHEMIA!! (although, we couldn't quite find a spot for diuretics)*

Constipation-inducing drugs
Opioids
Laxatives (osmotic agents, bisacodyl)
Oral contraceptives
NSAIDS

Immunomodulators
Serotoninergic drugs (alosetron, tegaserod)
Chemotherapeutic drugs (R-CHOP, taxanes, cisplatin)
Hormonal therapies (estrogen replacement)
Ergot alkaloids
Methamphetamine
Immunosuppressants (cyclosporin, tacrolimus)
Antibiotic-associated colitis

When CI is suspected, like in this case, you need to get to work with an expedited diagnostic workup. The ACG guidelines recommend a comprehensive set of labs. Key tests include albumin, amylase, a complete blood count, and a comprehensive electrolyte panel. It's also essential to measure creatine kinase, lactate, and lactate dehydrogenase levels to assess tissue damage and metabolic status. Additionally, stool tests to rule out infectious causes are critical; these should include assays for *C. difficile* toxin, culture tests, and tests for ova and parasites. This thorough lab workup helps pinpoint the underlying issues and guides appropriate management of the patient with suspected CI.

CT scans can help rule out other serious conditions (like diverticulitis), suggest a CI diagnosis (sometimes...), and identify affected colon areas. Common CT findings for CI include segmental wall thickening, thumbprinting), and pericolonic fat stranding, with or without ascites. In advanced cases you might find pneumatosis coli, a very concerning sign shown in **Figure 3.16**. When pneumatosis is found it portends a poor prognosis and suggests risk of transmural ischemia.

However, these signs are not specific enough for a definitive diagnosis. Studies have shown that typical CT findings of colitis are often nonspecific, highlighting the importance of further diagnostic work-up in patients with abdominal pain. In fact, when your pre-test probability of CI is very high in someone with recent-onset bloody diarrhea, and the CT scan is unremarkable, that might even increase your suspicion of CI in the right circumstance—not decrease it—because CT changes might simply not yet be evident, a finding consistent with early phase CI. So, while CT is important in the acute setting, it should be interpreted in conjunction with clinical findings to guide appropriate management. Remember, we don't treat the scan. We treat the patient. Think about the whole picture with all your patients. Scans are only part of the picture.

Figure 3.16. *Pneumatosis coli evident in the right colon. Image source: Brennan Spiegel, MD, MSHS.*

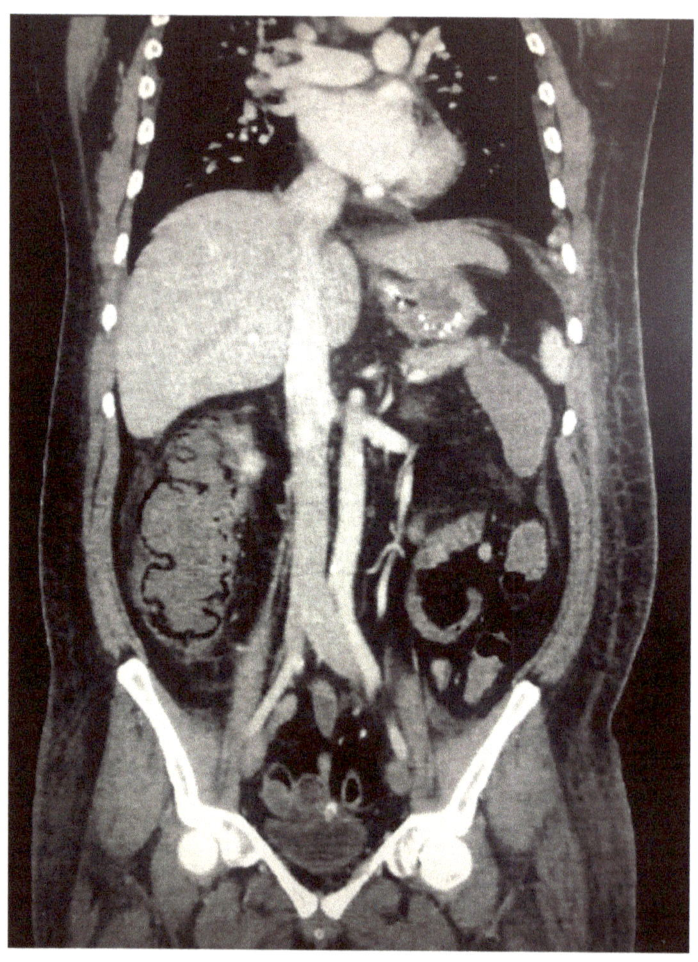

The clinical approach to CI depends on its severity. Patients with CI can present with varying degrees of severity, which dictates their management strategy. For those with mild CI, findings typically include segmental colitis not isolated to the right colon, without any major risk factors for poorer outcomes. These patients are usually managed with observation and supportive care.

Moderate CI involves more pronounced symptoms and up to three of the following risk factors: male gender, hypotension (systolic BP <90 mmHg), tachycardia (heart rate >100 bpm), abdominal pain without rectal bleeding, elevated BUN (>20 mg/dl), anemia (Hgb <12 g/dl), high LDH (>350 U/l), hyponatremia (serum sodium <136 mEq/l), leukocytosis (WBC >15 cells/cmm), or colonic mucosal ulceration identified via colonoscopy. Treatment for moderate CI includes addressing cardiovascular abnormalities, administering broad-spectrum antibiotics, and seeking surgical consultation.

Patients classified with **severe CI** exhibit more than three moderate criteria or critical signs such as peritoneal signs on physical examination, pneumatosis or portal venous gas on radiologic imaging, gangrene on colonoscopic examination, or pancolonic distribution or IRCI on imaging or colonoscopy. These patients need emergent surgical consultation, intensive care unit transfer, correction of cardiovascular abnormalities, broad-spectrum antibiotics, and likely will require surgery. **Figure 3.17** provides the full diagnostic and treatment algorithm from the ACG guidelines.

Alright, let's break down this flowchart for clinical assessment and management of CI while adding some essential clinical context:

Mild Disease. For patients presenting with typical symptoms of CI but without significant risk factors for poor outcomes, a CT of the abdomen and pelvis is recommended. If the CT is normal, go ahead with a colonoscopy to confirm the diagnosis. Remember, early colonoscopy (within 48 hours of presentation) should be performed to confirm. During the colonoscopy, minimal insufflation is advised to avoid exacerbating the condition by increasing colonic pressure and decreasing colon blood flow. It is preferable to use carbon dioxide

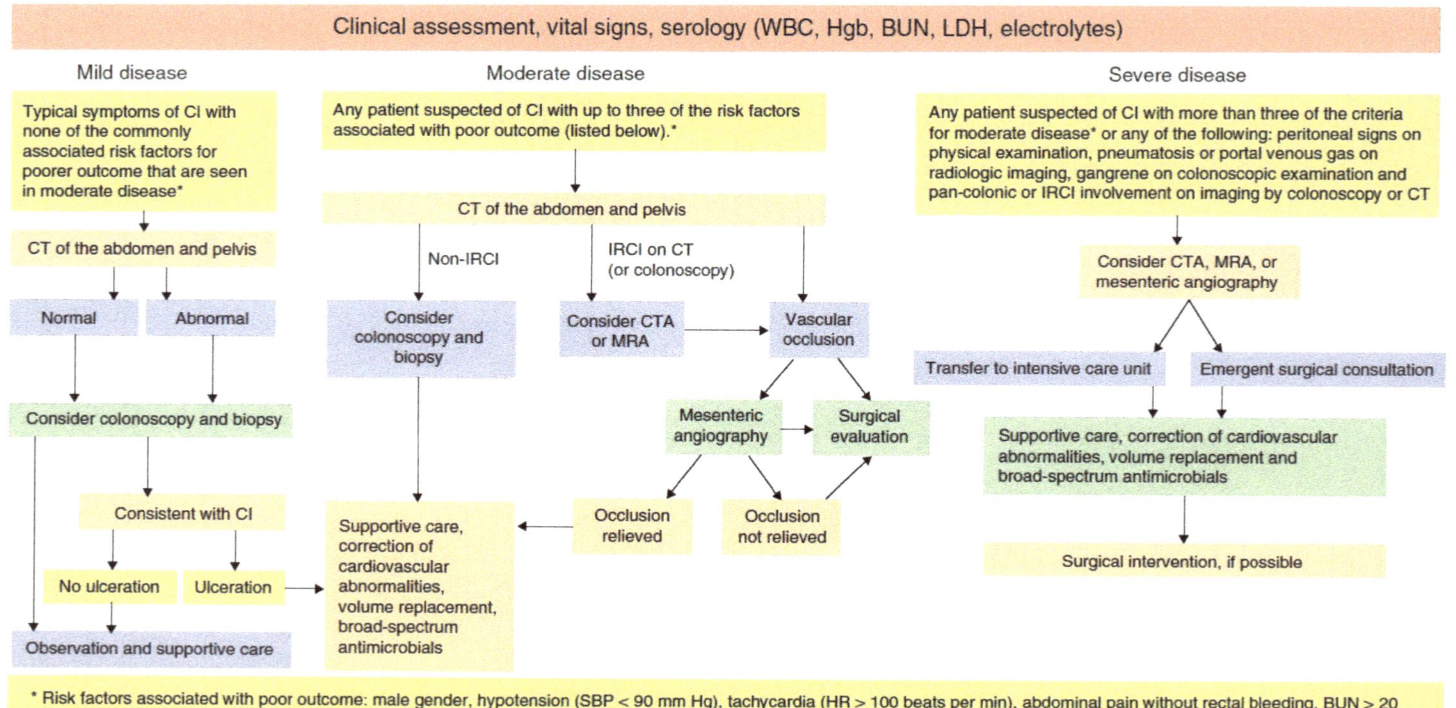

Figure 3.17. *Diagnostic and Treatment Algorithm for CI [Source: ACG Guidelines[137]*

rather than room air as the insufflating agent because carbon dioxide is rapidly absorbed and the gas actually increases colon blood flow. If no ulceration is found, the patient can be managed with observation and supportive care.

Moderate Disease. Patients having CI with up to three risk factors require a CT. If the CT shows non-isolated IRCI, a colonoscopy with biopsy is recommended. For those with more severe or suspicious findings on CT, further imaging with CTA or magnetic resonance angiography (MRA) may be warranted to evaluate for vascular occlusion, requiring mesenteric angiography or surgical evaluation. The colonoscopy in these cases should be limited to confirming the CT findings, and biopsies should be obtained except in cases of gangrene. Antibiotics should be considered for moderate or severe disease. Most cases of CI resolve spontaneously and do not require specific therapy.

Severe Disease: Patients with severe disease include those with more than three moderate disease risk factors, or any signs of severe pathology such as peritoneal signs, pneumatosis or portal venous gas on imaging, gangrene, or pancolonic involvement. For these patients, consider advanced imaging with CTA, MRA, or mesenteric angiography. These cases often require transfer to an ICU and emergent surgical consultation. Surgical intervention is especially critical if the patient shows signs of hypotension, tachycardia, and abdominal pain without rectal bleeding, or in the presence of gangrene. It's vital to note that colonoscopy should not be performed in patients with acute peritonitis or signs of perforation and should be halted if gangrene is found.

Overall, this algorithm emphasizes the importance of early and accurate diagnosis of CI, primarily through imaging and targeted colonoscopy, while also outlining the critical steps for managing varying severities of the condition, from supportive care in mild cases to surgical intervention in severe cases.

And with that, we have come to the end of *Guide to the Guidelines Volume 2.* We hope you found it useful. Stay tuned for Volume 3, which will cover all the pancreaticobiliary and liver guidelines from the ACG. In the meantime, test out your knowledge on GI bleeding with the next batch of questions, and feel free to circle back to Volume I to ensure you've also got those guidelines nailed down. See you again soon!

GI Bleeding Guidelines Quiz

1. Which of the following risk factors are not a part of the Glasgow-Blatchford score?

   a) Hemoglobin

   b) Systolic blood pressure

   c) Oxygen saturation

   d) BUN

   e) Melena

2. With a Glasgow-Blatchford score of 0 or 1, what percentage of patients would you expect that will not require a hospital-based intervention and can be safely discharged from the emergency department?

   a) 1%

   b) 20%

   c) 50%

   d) 70%

   e) 99%

3. An otherwise healthy 61-year-old man taking ibuprofen recently for knee pain presents with melena and indigestion without fatigue for the past 2 days to the emergency department. His BP is 118/69, HR 88, Hgb 13.6, BUN 12, creatinine 1.2. What is the most appropriate next step?

   a) Discharge home with outpatient follow-up

   b) Admit for observation and monitoring

   c) Admit with plan for EGD now

   d) Admit with plan for EGD within 24 hours

4. What is the threshold for transfusion for a patient with hemody-namically stable gastrointestinal hemorrhage with pre-existing car-diovascular disease?

   a) 6.0 g/dL
   b) 7.0 g/dL
   c) 8.0 g/dL
   d) 9.0 g/dL

5. An otherwise healthy 64-year-old woman taking naproxen for ar-thritis reports recent melena and fatigue and presents to the emer-gency department. Her abdominal exam is unremarkable. Her BP is 108/74, HR 96, hemoglobin 8.3, BUN 18, creatinine 1.1. What is the most appropriate next step?

   a) Nasogastric tube placement with aspiration to help determine source of bleeding
   b) Transfuse packed red blood cells
   c) Start intravenous proton pump inhibitor therapy
   d) Start intravenous fluid therapy
   e) Start intravenous prokinetic therapy

6. Empiric use of intravenous prokinetics in the management of UGI bleeding have been shown to help which of the following?

   a) Decrease ulcer rebleeding
   b) Decrease need for surgery
   c) Decrease mortality
   d) Decrease length of hospital stay
   e) Decrease transfusion requirement

7. What is the approximate rebleeding risk for an actively bleeding (oozing or spurting) peptic ulcer?

   a) 1%
   b) 1%
   c) 55%
   d) 99%

8. What is the approximate rebleeding risk for a peptic ulcer containing a non-bleeding visible vessel?

   a) 3%
   b) 13%
   c) 43%
   d) 93%

9. What is the approximate rebleeding risk of a peptic ulcer containing an adherent clot?

   a) 2%
   b) 22%
   c) 52%
   d) 92%

10. What is the approximate rebleeding risk for a peptic ulcer containing a flat pigmented spot?

   a) 1%
   b) 10%
   c) 50%
   d) 90%

11. What is the approximate rebleeding risk for a peptic ulcer with a clean base?

   a) 5%
   b) 25%
   c) 55%
   d) 95%

12. Which type of endoscopic therapy for peptic ulcer disease has shown the least evidence for achieving hemostasis?

   a) Probe contact electrocoagulation
   b) Argon plasma coagulation
   c) Absolute ethanol sclerotherapy
   d) Mechanical clip placement

13. You are doing an EGD for an inpatient with an upper GI bleed and find a gastric ulcer with an adherent clot. Which of the following is currently recommended by the evidence-based guidelines for this lesion?

a) Probe contact electrocoagulation with or without epinephrine injection

b) Mechanical clip placement with or without epinephrine injection

c) Observe without endoscopic therapy

d) Any of the above

14. You successfully achieved endoscopic hemostasis for an actively oozing 1 cm duodenal ulcer yesterday for an inpatient who initially presented with melena, hemoglobin 8.7 g/dL with normal vital signs. The patient has been placed on intravenous proton pump inhibitor therapy. You are now informed this morning that the patient has had new onset hematochezia with acute decrease in hemoglobin to 6.9 g/dL with BP 108/62 and HR 94. After volume resuscitation including blood transfusion, which of the following is the most appropriate next step in the management of this patient?

a) Arrange for EGD

b) Interventional Radiology consult for transcatheter arterial embolization

c) Surgery consult

d) Discontinue PPI due to lack of efficacy

15. Fluoroquinolone antibiotics have been linked to which of the following conditions?

a) Tendon rupture

b) Aortic dissection

c) *C. difficile* infection

d) Peripheral neuropathy

e) Drug interactions via the cytochrome P450 system

f) All of the above

16. Which of the following is not a criterion for acute, life-threatening
GI bleeding?

a) Decrease in hemoglobin > 5 g/dL
b) Requirement of ≥ 5 units packed red blood cell transfusion
c) Tachycardia > 120 beats per minute
d) Hypovolemic shock
e) Requirement of vasopressors

17. A 61-year-old woman on a factor Xa inhibiting DOAC is involved
in a motor vehicle accident and noted to have bleeding in multiple
sites throughout her body. She is hypotensive, placed on vasopressors and getting transfused in the trauma unit of the emergency
department. Alertly, the emergency department attending has ordered infusion of andexanet alfa and the bleeding ceases. Which
of the following DOACs would not show a favorable response to
this reversal agent?

a) Apixaban
b) Dagibatran
c) Rivoroxaban
d) Edoxaban

18. A 41-year-old patient develops life-threatening GI bleeding while
taking warfarin with INR 6.1. Which of the following is the most
appropriate reversal agent for this patient?

a) Vitamin K
b) Fresh frozen plasma
c) Prothrombin complex concentrate
d) Cryoprecipitate

19. A 68-year-old patient taking a DOAC presents with melena, normal vital signs and hemoglobin 11.3 g/dL. The DOAC has been
held. Which of the following is the best course of action in regard
to the current coagulopathy and management?

a) Supportive care and monitor
b) Provide the DOAC specific reversal agent
c) Provide prothombin complex concentrate
d) Provide fresh frozen plasma

20. A 79-year-old patient with a history significant for coronary artery stent placement 2 months ago with a drug-eluting stent on aspirin 81 mg daily and clopidogrel 75 mg daily develops severe, acute life-threatening GI bleeding. Complete blood count shows hemoglobin 6.8 g/dL and platelets 192K. You have arranged for intensive care unit admission, volume resuscitation and blood transfusion. In addition, you should also recommend platelet transfusion for this patient.

a) True

b) False

21. Acetylsalicylic acid (ASA) inhibits platelets via a COX-1 enzyme pathway.

a) True
b) False

22. Irreversible effects by medications on platelets last about 2 weeks.

a) True
b) False

23. COX-2 selective NSAIDs inhibit platelet function also.

a) True
b) False

24. There has been a demonstrated mortality benefit for early resumption of ASA after endoscopic hemostasis of bleeding peptic ulcers.

a) True
b) False

25. Bare-metal coronary stents require a longer duration of dual anti-platelet therapy than drug-eluting coronary stents.

a) True
b) False

26. When it comes to managing GI bleeding, the heart is more important than the gut.

a) True

 b) False

27. Which of the following is not a CHA$_2$DS$_2$-VASc risk factor for thromboembolism? Age >40 at diagnosis

a) Congestive heart failure
b) Advanced age
c) Diabetes mellitus
d) Hypertension
e) Male gender
f) History of stroke

28. Which of the following variables of the Oakland score for prognosticating lower GI hemorrhage does not increase the risk requiring a hospital-based intervention?

a) Advanced age
b) Female gender
c) History of previous lower GI bleeding
d) Positive for blood on digital rectal examination
e) Tachycardia
f) Hypotension
g) Anemia

29. A 64-year-old man with history of stroke, now with full recovery on ASA 81mg daily presents with hematochezia for 2 days without abdominal pain prior to arrival to the emergency department today. BP 118/69, HR 94. Abdomen is soft and non-tender. Hgb 11.2 g/dL. He had sigmoid diverticulosis and no polyps noted on screening colonoscopy last year. He has been admitted to the hospital this evening without further bleeding. Which of the following if the most appropriate next step?

a) Hold ASA and start bowel preparation for colonoscopy in the morning
b) Continue ASA and start bowel preparation for colonoscopy in the morning
c) Hold ASA and monitor for further bleeding
d) Continue ASA and monitor for further bleeding
e) CT angiography now

30. Which of the following is the most common etiology of hematochezia causing hospitalization?

    a) Colonic neoplasia
    b) Benign colonic ulcers
    c) Arteriovenous malformations
    d) Diverticular hemorrhage
    e) Brisk upper GI bleeding

31. A 79-year-old woman with hypertension, hyperlipidemia and re-
mote history of myocardial infarction, who cannot recall her current
medication list, presents to the emergency department with severe
hematochezia. Vitals show BP 106/69 and HR 102. Which of the
following is the most appropriate initial strategy in management?

    a) Volume resuscitation
    b) CT angiogram
    c) Arrange for immediate colonoscopy
    d) IR consult for transcatheter arteriography with embolization

32. In the patient noted above, resuscitation with IV fluids and packed
red blood cell (PRBC) transfusion has been undertaken and an
EGD is negative for bleeding. You are alerted that she is still passing
several large bloody bowel movements. What is the next most appropriate step in management?

    a) Arrange for immediate colonoscopy
    b) IR consult for transcatheter arteriography with embolization
    c) CT angiogram
    d) Small bowel video capsule endoscopy

33. For best chance to demonstrate active bleeding via contrast
extravasation, a CT angiogram should be performed in which of
the following timeframes after a bloody bowel movement?

    a) Within 4 hours
    b) Within 24 hours
    c) Within 48 hours
    d) Timing does not make a difference

34. After a CT angiogram demonstrates contrast extravasation, when should our IR colleagues perform transcatheter arteriography with targeted embolization for the best chance to achieve hemostasis

a) Within 90 minutes
b) Within 240 minutes
c) Within 480 minutes
d) Timing does not make a difference

35. Which endoscopic modality is the most optimal strategy for management of a patient with AVM bleeding?

a) Epinephrine injection
b) Argon plasma coagulation
c) Contact probe electrocoagulation
d) Mechanical clip placement

36. A 45-year-old woman has an outpatient screening colonoscopy with snare polypectomy for an 18 mm polyp in the proximal transverse colon at an endoscopic center of excellence in a tertiary hospital. The next day she promptly returns to the emergency department at the hospital due to symptomatic anemia from severe hematochezia. She is getting resuscitation in the ED and requires PRBC transfu-sion. What is the best management option for hemostasis?

a) Urgent colonoscopy with a split dose bowel preparation and clip placement
b) Transcatheter arteriography with embolization
c) Observation and supportive care
d) Surgery consultation

37. A patient on warfarin with a supratherapeutic INR is admitted to the hospital due to active GI bleeding. What INR range is considered safe and effective for endoscopic hemostasis?

a) INR ≤ 4.5
b) INR ≤ 3.5
c) INR ≤ 2.5
d) Any INR is considered safe and effective

38. Which of the following endoscopic therapies is effective to achieve hemostasis for an actively bleeding colonic diverticulum?

a) Endoscopic band ligation
b) Through-the-scope clip placement
c) Contact probe coagulation
d) All of the above

39. A 78-year-old man with history of diverticular hemorrhage five years ago presents with marked hematochezia and is promptly admitted to the hospital. He undergoes resuscitation. A colonoscopy is performed and a sigmoid diverticulum with stigmata of recent hemorrhage is found. If contact probe electrocoagulation is performed for endoscopic hemostasis, then which location on the diverticulum is suitable for this type of therapy?

a) Rim or neck of the diverticulum
b) Base of the diverticulum
c) Any location on the diverticulum is fine
d) None of the above

40. Isolated right-sided colon ischemia is typically characterized by which of the following, in comparison to left-sided colon ischemia:

a) Less abdominal pain
b) Less rectal bleeding
c) Lower mortality
d) Less underlying cardiovascular disease

Answers to GI Bleeding Guidelines Quiz

1.	C	21.	A
2.	E	22.	B
3.	A	23.	B
4.	C	24.	A
5.	D	25.	B
6.	D	26.	A
7.	C	27.	E
8.	C	28.	B
9.	B	29.	D
10.	B	30.	D
11.	A	31.	A
12.	B	32.	C
13.	D	33.	A
14.	A	34.	A
15.	F	35.	B
16.	C	36.	A
17.	B	37.	C
18.	C	38.	D
19.	A	39.	A
20.	B	40.	B

Acknowledgments

We thank the authors of the ACG guidelines covered in this book who provided expert review on their sections: William D. Chey, MD, FACG; Gary Lichtenstein, MD, FACG, David Rubin, MD, FACG; Colin Howden, MD, FACG; Colleen Kelly, MD, FACG; Mark Riddle, MD; Loren Laine, MD, FACG; Grigorios Leontiadis, MD, PhD, FACG; Neil Sengupta, MD, FACG; and Lawrence Brandt, MD, MACG. In addition, we thank the ACG Board of Trustees and Practice Parameters Committee for their continued work on developing guidelines and supporting the GI community. Lastly, we thank the ACG editorial team for their production and editing work on this book: Claire Neumann, Neen LeMaster, and Angélica Bermúdez .

Personal Dedications

H.K.: To my grandfather, Kasanji, who provided countless uplifting words of inspiration, encouragement and motivation. His unfulfilled dreams for higher education were never lost upon me. *Iamque opus exegi.* Om Shanti Shanti Shanti.

B.S.: To my mother-in-law, Vivian Turner, for her unwavering support of our family.

Authors' Note

We wrote this book using good old-fashioned human intelligence. After writing the text, we employed Chat GPT-4o to help copyedit the passages. We believe it remains important that humans—not computers—write for other humans, but also recognize benefits of AI to support editing of original text written by humans.

MEET THE AUTHORS

Brennan Spiegel, MD, MSHS, FACG

Dr. Spiegel is the Dorothy and George Gourrich Chair in Digital Health Ethics at Cedars-Sinai, Founding Director of the Cedars-Sinai Master's Degree Program in Health Science Systems, and an ACG Governor for Southern California. He is the immediate past Editor-in-Chief for *The American Journal of Gastroenterology* and inaugural Editor-in-Chief for the *Journal of Medical Extended Reality*. Dr. Spiegel has published widely in the fields of health services research, digital health, use of virtual reality in medicine, and clinical gastroenterology across a range of topics. Together with Dr. Karsan, he also wrote the "Acing the GI Board Exam" series of books.

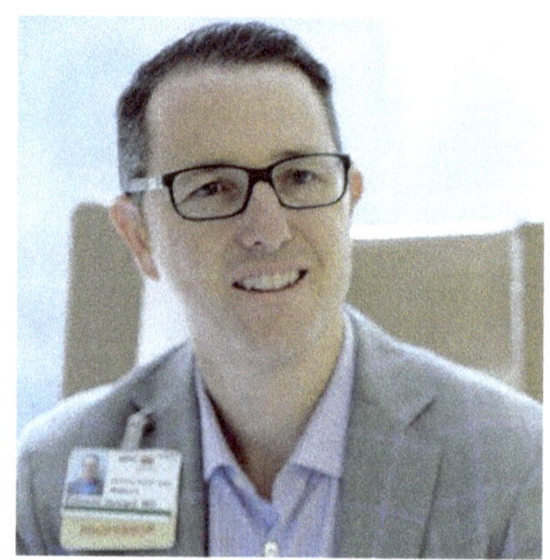

Hetal A. Karsan, FACG, AGAF, FASGE, FAASLD, FACP

Dr. Karsan is the Chair of Medical Education and Executive Committee Member for United Digestive, while also being Adjunct Professor of Medicine in the Division of Digestive Diseases at Emory University. In addition, he serves as the Chair of the Credentials Committee, International Governor, and Governor of Georgia for the ACG. He is the immediate past Editor of the Red Section and Associate Editor for *The American Journal of Gastroenterology*. He has practiced for more than twenty years in both private and academic settings, while actively maintaining board certifications in Gastroenterology, Transplant Hepatology and Internal Medicine. Collaborating with Dr. Spiegel, he wrote the "Acing the GI Board Exam" series of textbooks.

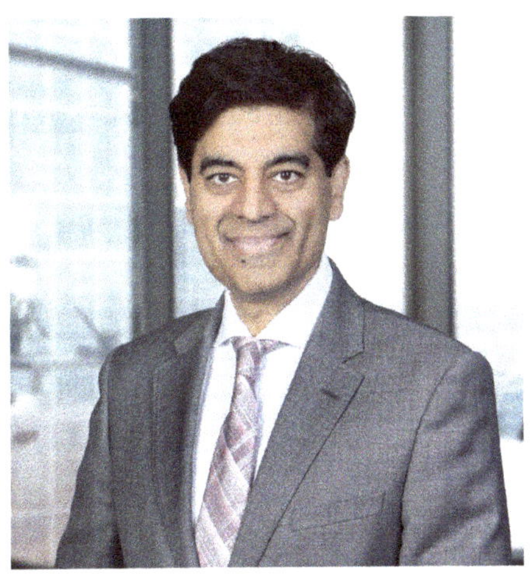

REFERENCES

1.   Lichtenstein GR, Loftus E, Isaacs K, et al. ACG clinical guideline: Management of Crohn's disease in adults. Am J Gastroenterol 2018;113:481-517

2.   Center for Disese Control (CDC). IBD Facts and Stats. Accessed September 12th 2024. Website: https://www.cdc.gov/inflammatory-bowel-disease/php/facts-stats/index.html#:~:text=U.S.%20prevalence%20of%20inflammatory%20bowel,health%20care%20costs%20are%20rising.

3.   Van Rheenen PF, Van de Vijver E, Fidler V. Faecal calprotectin for screening of patients with suspected inflammatory bowel disease: Diagnostic meta-analysis. BMJ 2010;341:c3369.

4.   Vermeire S, Van Assche G, Rutgeerts P. C-reactive protein as a marker for inflammatory bowel disease. Inflamm Bowel Dis 2004;10:661-665.

5.   Mitsuyama K, Niwa M, Takedatsu H et al. Antibody markers in the diagnosis of inflammatory bowel disease. World J Gastroenterol 2016;22:1304-1310.

6.   Byrne M, Power D, Keeling A et al. Combined terminal ileoscopy and biopsy is superior to small bowel follow-through in detecting terminal ileal pathology. Dig Liv Dis 2004;36:147-152.

7.   Dionisio P, Gurudu S, Leighton J et al. Capsule endoscopy has a significantly higher diagnostic yield in patients with suspected and established small-bowel Crohn's disease: a meta-analysis. Am J Gastroenterol 2010;105:1240-1248.

8.   Solem C, Loftus EJ, Fletcher J et al. Small-bowel imaging in Crohn's disease: a prospective, blinded, 4-way comparison trial. Gastrointest Endosc 2008;68:255-266.

9.   Church P, Turner D, Feldman B et al. Systematic review with meta-analysis: magnetic resonance enterography signs for the detection of inflammation and intestinal damage in Crohn's disease. Aliment Pharmacol Ther 2015;41:153-166.

10.   Samuel S, Bruining D, Loftus E, Jr et al. Endoscopic skipping of the distal terminal ileum in Crohn's disease can lead to negative results from ileocolonoscopy. Clin Gastroenterol Hepatol 2012;10:1253-1259.

11.   Van Der Sloot KW, Joshi AD, Bellavance DR et al. Visceral adiposity, genetic susceptibility, and risk of complications among individuals with Crohn's disease. Inflamm Bowel Dis 2017;23:82-88.

12.   Van Assche G, Dignass A, Panes J et al. The second European evidence-based consensus on the diagnosis and management of Crohn's disease: definitions and diagnosis. J Crohns Colitis 2010;4:7-27.

13.   Winship DH, Summers RW, Singleton JW, Best WR, Becktel JM, Lenk LF, Kern F Jr. National Cooperative Crohn's Disease Study: study design and conduct of the study. Gastroenterology 1979;77:829–842.

14.   Boschetti G, Laidet M, Moussata D et al. Levels of fecal calprotectin are associated with the severity of postoperative endoscopic recurrence in asymptomatic patients with Crohn's disease. Am J Gastroenterol 2015;110:865-872.

15.   Magro F, Rodrigues-Pinto E, Santos-Antunes J et al. High C-reactive protein in Crohn's disease patients predicts nonresponse to infliximab treatment. J Crohns Colitis 2014;8:129-136.

16.   Tielbeek J, Löwenberg M, Bipat S et al. Serial magnetic resonance imaging for monitoring medical therapy effects in Crohn's disease. Inflamm Bowel Dis 2013;19:1943-1950.

17.   Schwartz D, White C, Wise P et al. Use of endoscopic ultrasound to guide combination medical and surgical therapy for patients with Crohn's perianal fistulas. Inflamm Bowel Dis 2005;11:727-732.

18.   Takeuchi K, Smale S, Premchand P et al. Prevalence and mechanism of nonsteroidal anti-inflammatory drug-induced clinical relapse in patients with inflammatory bowel disease. Clin Gastroenterol Hepatol 2006;4:196-202.

19.   Singh S, Graff L, Bernstein C. Do NSAIDs, antibiotics, infections, or stress trigger flares in IBD? Am J Gastroenterol 2008;104:1298-1313.

20.   Kuenzig ME, Lee SM, Eksteen B et al. Smoking influences the need for surgery in patients with the inflammatory bowel diseases: a systematic review and meta-analysis incorporating disease duration. BMC Gastroenterol 2016;16:143.

21.   Aberra F, Brensinger C, Bilker W et al. Antibiotic Use and the Risk of Flare of Inflammatory Bowel Disease. Clin Gastroenterol Hepatol 2005;3:459-465.

22.   Gaines L, Slaughter J, Horst S et al. Association between affective-cognitive symptoms of depression and exacerbation of Crohn's disease. Am J Gastroenterol 2016;111:864-870.

23.   Tremaine WJ, Hanauer SB, Katz S et al. Budesonide CIR capsules (once or twice daily divided-dose) in active Crohn's disease: a randomized placebo-controlled study in the United States. Am J Gastroenterol 2002;97:1748-1754.

24.   Ford A, Kane S, Khan K et al. Efficacy of 5-aminosalicylates in Crohn's disease: systematic review and meta-analysis. Am J Gastroenterol 2011;106:617-629.

25.   Khan KJ, Ullman TA, Ford AC et al. Antibiotic therapy in inflammatory bowel disease: a systematic review and meta-analysis. Am J Gastroenterol 2011;106:661-673.

26.   Rutgeerts P, Van Assche G, Vermeire S et al. Ornidazole for prophylaxis of postoperative Crohn's disease recurrence: a randomized, double-blind, placebo-controlled trial. Gastroenterology 2005;128:856-861.

27.   Prantera C, Lochs H, Grimaldi M et al. Rifaximin-extended intestinal release induces remission in patients with moderately active Crohn's disease. Gastroenterology 2012;142:473-481; e4.

28.   Borgaonkar MR, MacIntosh DG, Fardy JM. A meta-analysis of antimycobacterial therapy for Crohn's disease. Am J Gastroenterol 2000;95:725-729.

29.   Lewis JD, Sandler RS, Brotherton C, et al. A Randomized Trial Comparing the Specific Carbohydrate Diet to a Mediterranean Diet in Adults With Crohn's Disease Gastroenterology 2021;161:837 - 852

30.   Colombel JF, Sandborn WJ, Reinisch W et al. Infliximab, azathioprine, or combination therapy for Crohn's disease. N Engl J Med 2010;362:1383-1395.

31.   Hazlewood GS, Rezaie A, Borman M et al. Comparative effectiveness of immunosuppressants and biologics for inducing and maintaining remission in Crohn's disease: a network meta-analysis. Gastroenterology 2015;148:344-354.e5; quiz e14-5.

32.   Parks AG, Gordon PH, Hardcastle JD. A classification of fistula-in-ano. British J of Surgery 1976;63:1-12.

33.   Nguyen GC, Loftus EV Jr., Hirano I et al. American Gastroenterological Association Institute Guideline on the management of Crohn's disease after surgical resection. Gastroenterology 2017;152:271-275.

34.   Singh S, Garg SK, Pardi DS et al. Comparative efficacy of pharmacologic interventions in preventing relapse of Crohn's disease after surgery: a systematic review and network meta-analysis. Gastroenterology 2015;148:64-76.e2

35.   Hupé M, Pereira B, Mathieu, et al. Network meta-analysis comparing efficacy between biologics and conventional therapies to prevent endoscopic postoperative recurrence in patients with Crohn's disease. Journal of Crohn's and Colitis 2024;i1197, Supplement

36.   Rubin DT, Ananthakrishnan AN, Siegel CA, et al. ACG clinical guideline: ulcerative colitis in adults. Am J Gastroenterol 2019;114:384-413

37.   Walmsley RS, Ayres RC, Pounder RE, et al. A Simple Clinical Colitis Activity Index. Gut 1998;43:29–32.

38.   Ford AC, Achkar JP, Khan KJ, et al. Efficacy of 5-aminosalicylates in ulcerative colitis: Systematic review and meta-analysis. Am J Gastroenterol 2011;106:601–16.

39.   Marshall JK, Thabane M, Steinhart AH, et al. Rectal 5-aminosalicylic acid for induction of remission in ulcerative colitis. Cochrane Database Syst Rev 2010:CD004115.

40.   Ford AC, Khan KJ, Achkar JP, et al. Efficacy of oral vs topical, or combined oral and topical 5-aminosalicylates, in ulcerative colitis: Systematic review and meta-analysis. Am J Gastroenterol 2012;107:167–76; author reply 177.

41.   Ford AC, Bernstein CN, Khan KJ, et al. Glucocorticosteroid therapy in inflammatory bowel disease: Systematic review and meta-analysis. Am J Gastroenterol 2011;106:590–9; quiz 600.

42.   Rubin DT, Cohen RD, Sandborn WJ, et al. Budesonide multimatrix is efficacious for mesalamine-refractory, mild to moderate ulcerative colitis: A randomised, placebo-controlled trial. J Crohns Colitis 2017;11:785–91.

43.   Sandborn WJ, Travis S, Moro L, et al. Once-daily budesonide MMX(R) extended-release tablets induce remission in patients with mild to moderate ulcerative colitis: Results from the CORE I study. Gastroenterology 2012;143:1218–26.e1–2.

44.   Danese S, Fiorino G, Peyrin-Biroulet L, et al. Biological agents for moderately to severely active ulcerative colitis: A systematic review and network meta-analysis. Ann Intern Med 2014;160:704–11.

45.   Stidham RW, Lee TC, Higgins PD, et al. Systematic review with network meta-analysis: The efficacy of anti-tumour necrosis factor-alpha agents for the treatment of ulcerative colitis. Aliment Pharmacol Ther 2014;39:660–71.

46.   Feagan BG, Rubin DT, Danese S, et al. Efficacy of vedolizumab induction and maintenance therapy in patients with ulcerative colitis, regardless of prior exposure to tumor necrosis factor antagonists. Clin Gastroenterol Hepatol 2017;15:229–39.

47.   Sandborn WJ, Su C, Sands BE, et al. Tofacitinib as induction and maintenance therapy for ulcerative colitis. N Engl J Med 2017;376:1723–36.

48.   Lutgens MW, van Oijen MG, van der Heijden GJ, et al. Declining risk of colorectal cancer in inflammatory bowel disease: An updated meta-analysis of population-based cohort studies. Inflamm Bowel Dis 2013;19:789–99.

49.   Rubio-Tapia A, Hill ID, Semrad C, et al. ACG guidelines update: diagnosis and management of celiac disease. Am J Gastroenterol 2023;118:59-76

50.   Irvine AJ, Chey WD, Ford AC. Screening for celiac disease in irritable bowel syndrome: an updated systematic review and meta-analysis. Am J Gastroenterol. 2017;112:65-76

51.   Lebwohl B, Kapel RC, Neugut AI, et al. Adherence to biopsy guidelines increases celiac disease diagnosis. Gastrointest Endosc 2011;74(1):103–9.

52.   Chey WD, Howden CW, Moss SF, et al. ACG clinical practice guidelines on the treatment of *Helicobacter pylori* infection. Am J Gastroenterol 2024; 119:1730-53.

53.   Li Y, Choi H, Leung K, et al. Global prevalence of *Helicobacter pylori* infection between 1980 and 2022: a systematic review and meta-analysis. Lancet Gastroenterol Hepatol 2023;8:553-564.

54.   Moayyedi P, Lacy B, Andrews C, et al. ACG and CAG clinical guideline: management of dyspepsia. Am J Gastroenterol. 2017;112:988-1013.

55.   Alsamman MA, Vecchio EC, Shawwa K, et al. Retrospective analysis confirms tetracycline quadruple as best *Helicobacter pylori* Regimen in the USA. Dig Dis Sci 2019;64:2893-2898.

56.   Ho JJC, Navarro M, Sawyer K, et al. *Helicobacter pylori* Antibiotic Resistance in the United States Between 2011 and 2021: A Systematic Review and Meta-Analysis. Am J Gastroenterol 2022;117:1221-1230.

57.   Rokkas T, Gisbert JP, Malfertheiner P, et al. Comparative effectiveness of multiple different first-line treatment regimens for *Helicobacter pylori* infection: A network meta-analysis. Gastroenterology 2021;161:495-507 e4.

58.   Laine L, Sharma P, Mulford DJ, et al. Pharmacodynamics and pharmacokinetics of the potassium-competitive acid blocker vonoprazan and the proton pump inhibitor lansoprazole in US subjects. Am J Gastroenterol 2022;117:1158-1161.

59.   Chey WD, Megraud F, Laine L, et al. Vonoprazan Triple and Dual Therapy for *Helicobacter pylori* Infection in the United States and Europe: Randomized Clinical Trial. Gastroenterology 2022;163:608-619.

60.   Qian HS, Li WJ, Dang YN, et al. Ten-Day Vonoprazan-Amoxicillin Dual Therapy as a First-Line Treatment of *Helicobacter pylori* Infection Compared With Bismuth-Containing Quadruple Therapy. Am J Gastroenterol 2023;118:627-634.

61.   Kelly, CR, Fischer M, Allegretti JR, et al. ACG clinical guidelines: prevention, diagnosis, and treatment of *Clostridioides difficle*. Am J Gastroenterol 2021;116:1124-1147.

62.   O'Horo JC, Jones A, Sternke M, et al. Molecular techniques for diagnosis of *Clostridium difficile* infection: Systematic review and meta-analysis. Mayo Clin Proc 2012;87:643–51.

63.   O'Horo JC, Jones A, Sternke M, et al. Molecular techniques for diagnosis of *Clostridium difficile* infection: Systematic review and meta-analysis. Mayo Clin Proc 2012;87:643–51.

64.   Cohen SH, Gerding DN, Johnson S, et al. Clinical practice guidelines for *Clostridium difficile* infection in adults: 2010 update by the society for healthcare epide-

miology of America (SHEA) and the infectious diseases society of America (IDSA). Infect Control Hosp Epidemiol 2010;31:431–55.

65.   Stevens VW, Shoemaker HE, Jones MM, et al. Validation of the SHEA/IDSA severity criteria to predict poor outcomes among inpatients and outpatients with *Clostridioides difficile* infection. Infect Control Hosp Epidemiol 2020;41:510–6.

66.   Crook DW, Walker AS, Kean Y, et al. Fidaxomicin versus vancomycin for Clostridium difficile infection: meta-analysis of pivotal randomized controlled trials. Clin Infect Dis 2012;55(Suppl 2):S93–103.

67.   Beinortas T, Burr NE, Wilcox MH, et al. Comparative efficacy of treatments for Clostridium difficile infection: A systematic review and network meta-analysis. Lancet Infect Dis 2018;18:1035–44.

68.   Watt M, Dinh A, Le Monnier A, et al. Cost-effectiveness analysis on the use of fidaxomicin and vancomycin to treat Clostridium difficile infection in France. J Med Econ 2017;20:678–86.

69.   Fekety R, Silva J, Kauffman C, et al. Treatment of antibiotic-associated Clostridium difficile colitis with oral vancomycin: Comparison of two dosage regimens. Am J Med 1989;86:15–9.

70.   Agrawal M, Aroniadis OC, Brandt LJ, et al. The long-term efficacy and safety of fecal microbiota transplant for recurrent, severe, and complicated Clostridium difficile infection in 146 elderly individuals. J Clin Gastroenterol 2016;50:403–7.

71.   Zainah H, Hassan M, Shiekh-Sroujieh L, et al. Intestinal microbiota transplantation, a simple and effective treatment for severe and refractory Clostridium difficile infection. Dig Dis Sci 2015;60:181–5.

72.   Cammarota G, Ianiro G, Magalini S, et al. Decrease in surgery for Clostridium difficile infection after starting a program to transplant fecal microbiota. Ann Intern Med 2015;163:487–8.

73.   van Nood E, Vrieze A, Nieuwdorp M, et al. Duodenal infusion of donor feces for recurrent Clostridium difficile. N Engl J Med 2013;368:407–15.

74.   Kelly CR, Khoruts A, Staley C, et al. Effect of fecal microbiota transplantation on recurrence in multiply recurrent Clostridium difficile infection: A randomized trial. Ann Intern Med 2016;165:609–16.

75.   Tariq R, Singh S, Gupta A, et al. Association of gastric acid suppression with recurrent Clostridium difficile infection: A systematic review and meta-analysis. JAMA Intern Med 2017;177:784–91.

76.   Moayyedi P, Eikelboom JW, Bosch J, et al. Safety of proton pump inhibitors based on a large, multi-year, randomized trial of patients receiving rivaroxaban or aspirin. Gastroenterology 2019;157:682–91.e2.

77.   Singh H, Nugent Z, Yu BN, et al. Higher incidence of Clostridium difficile infection among individuals with inflammatory bowel disease. Gastroenterology 2017;153:430–8.e2.

78.   Qazi T, Amaratunga T, Barnes EL, et al. The risk of inflammatory bowel disease flares after fecal microbiota transplantation: Systematic review and meta-analysis. Gut Microbes 2017;8:574–88.

79.   Allegretti JR, Kelly CR, Grinspan A, et al. Outcomes of fecal microbiota transplantation in patients with inflammatory bowel diseases and recurrent *Clostridioides difficile* infection. Gastroenterology 2020;159:1982–4.

80.   Riddle MS, DuPont HL, Bradley C. ACG clinical guidelie: diagnosis, treatment, and prevention of acute diarrheal infections in adults. Am J Gastroenterol. 2016;111:602-622

81.   Laine, L, Barkun AN, Saltzman JR, Martel M, Leontiadis GI. ACG Clinical Guideline: Upper Gastrointestinal and Ulcer Bleeding. Am J Gastroenterol. 2021 May 1;116(5):899-917.

82.   Blatchford O, Murray WR, Blatchford M. A risk score to predict need for treatment for upper-gastrointestinal haemorrhage. Lancet 2000;356:1318–21.

83.   Laursen SB, Dalton HR, Murray IA, et al. Performance of new thresholds of the Glasgow Blatchford score in managing patients with upper gastrointestinal bleeding. Clin Gastroenterol Hepatol 2015;13:115–21.

84.   Carson JL, Stanworth SJ, Guyatt G, et al. Red Blood Cell Transfusion: 2023 AABB International Guidelines. JAMA. 2023 Nov 21;330(19):1892-1902.

85.   Villanueva C, Colomo A, Bosch A, et al. Transfusion strategies for acute upper gastrointestinal bleeding. N Engl J Med 2013;368:11–21.

86.   Rockey DC, Ahn C, de Melo SW. Randomized pragmatic trial of nasogastric tube placement in patients with upper gastrointestinal tract bleeding. J Investig Med 2017; 65: 759–764.

87.   Rahman R, Nguyen DL, Sohail U, et al. Pre-endoscopic erythromycin administration in upper gastrointestinal bleeding: An updated meta-analysis and systematic review. Ann Gastroenterol 2016;29:312–7.

88.   Barkun AN, Bardou M, Martel M, et al. Prokinetics in acute upper GI bleeding: A meta-analysis. Gastrointest Endosc 2010;72:1138–45.

89.   Daram SR, Garretson R. Erythromycin is preferable to metoclopramide as a prokinetic in acute upper GI bleeding. Gastrointest Endosc 2011;74: 234.

90.   Barkun AN, Bardou M, Martel M, et al. Response. Gastrointest Endosc 2011;74:234–5.

91.   Vimonsuntirungsri T, Thungsuk R, Nopjaroonsri P, et al. The Efficacy of Metoclopramide for Gastric Visualization by Endoscopy in Patients With Active Upper Gastrointestinal Bleeding: Double-Blind Randomized Controlled Trial. Am J Gastroenterol. 2024 May 1;119(5):846-855.

92.   Manupeeraphant P, Wanichagool D, Songlin T, et al. Intravenous metoclopramide for increasing endoscopic mucosal visualization in patients with acute upper gastrointestinal bleeding: a multicenter, randomized, double-blind, controlled trial. Sci Rep. 2024 Mar 31;14(1):7598.

93.   Lau JY, Leung WK, Wu JC, et al. Omeprazole before endoscopy in patients with gastrointestinal bleeding. N Engl J Med 2007;356:1631–40.

94.   Laine L, McQuaid KR. Endoscopic therapy for bleeding ulcers: An evidence-based approach based on meta-analyses of randomized controlled trials. Clin Gastroenterol Hepatol 2009;7:33–47.

95.   Orpen-Palmer J, Stanley AJ. Update on the management of upper gastrointestinal bleeding. BMJ Med. 2022; Sep 28;1(1)

96.   National Institute for Health and Care Excellence. Acute Upper Gastrointestinal Bleeding in Over 16s: Management. CG141. 2012.

97.   Gralnek IM, Stanley AJ, Morris AJ, et al. Endoscopic diagnosis and management of nonvariceal upper gastrointestinal hemorrhage (NVUGIH): European Society of Gastrointestinal Endoscopy (ESGE) Guideline - Update 2021. Endoscopy. 2021 Mar;53(3):300-332.

98.   Spiegel BM, Vakil NB, Ofman JJ. Endoscopy for acute nonvariceal upper gastrointestinal tract hemorrhage: is sooner better? A systematic review. Arch Intern Med. 2001;161:1393-404

99.   Lau JYW, Yu Y, Tang RSY, et al. Timing of endoscopy for acute upper gastrointestinal bleeding. N Engl J Med 2020;382:1299–308.

100. Forrest JA, Finlayson ND, Shearman DJ. Endoscopy in gastroinestial bleeding. Lancet. 1974 Aug 17;2(7877):394-7.

101. Laine L , Peterson WL . Bleeding peptic ulcer . N Engl J Med 1994 ; 331:717 – 727.

102. Laine L, Jensen DM. Management of patients with ulcer bleeding. Am J Gastroenterol. 2012 Mar;107(3):345-360.

103. Schmidt A, Golder S, Goetz M, et al. Over-the-scope clips are more effective than standard endoscopic therapy for patients with recurrent bleeding of peptic ulcers. Gastroenterology 2018;155:674–86.

104.   Cheng HC, Chung-Tai W, Chang WL, et al. Double oral esomeprazole after a 3-day intravenous esomeprazole infusion reduces recurrent peptic ulcer bleeding in high-risk patients: a randomised controlled study. Gut 2014;63:1864–72.

105.   Laine L, Jensen DM. Management of patients with ulcer bleeding. Am J Gastroenterol 2012;107:345–60.

106.   Lau JY, Sung JJ, Lam YH, et al. Endoscopic retreatment compared with surgery in patients with recurrent bleeding after initial endoscopic control of bleeding ulcers. N Engl J Med 1999;340:751–6.

107.   Tarasconi A, Baiocchi GL, Pattonieri V, et al. Transcatheter arterial embolization versus surgery for refractory non-variceal upper gastrointestinal bleeding: A meta-analysis. World J Emerg Surg 2019; 14:3.

108.   Sverden E, Mattsson F, Lindstrom D, et al. Transcatheter arterial embolization compared with surgery for uncontrolled peptic ulcer bleeding: A population-based cohort study. Ann Surg 2019;269:304–9.

109.   Abraham NS, Barkun AN, Sauer BG, Douketis J, Laine L, Noseworthy PA, Telford JJ, Leontiadis GI. American College of Gastroenterology-Canadian Association of Gastroenterology Clinical Practice Guideline: Management of Anticoagulants and Antiplatelets During Acute Gastrointestinal Bleeding and the Periendoscopic Period. Am J Gastroenterol. 2022 Apr 1;117(4):542-558.

110.   Baggio D., Ananda-Rajah M.R. Fluoroquinolone antibiotics and adverse events. Aust. Prescr. 2021; 44:161–164.

111.   Jones C.B., Fugate S.E. Levofloxacin and Warfarin Interaction. Ann. Pharmacother. 2002; 36:1554–1557.

112.   Mehran R, Rao SV, Bhatt DL, et al. Standardized bleeding definitions for cardiovascular clinical trials: A consensus report from the Bleeding Academic Research Consortium. Circulation 2011;123(23):2736–47.

113.   Moustafa F, Stehouwer A, Kamphuisen P, et al. Management and outcome of major bleeding in patients receiving vitamin K antagonists for venous thromboembolism. Thromb Res 2018;171:74–80.

114.   Barkun AN, Douketis J, Noseworthy PA, Laine L, Telford JJ, Abraham NS. Management of Patients on Anticoagulants and Antiplatelets During Acute Gastrointestinal Bleeding and the Peri-Endoscopic Period: A Clinical Practice Guideline Dissemination Tool. Am J Gastroenterol. 2022 Apr 1;117(4):513-519.

115.   Levine GN, Bates ER, Bittl JA, et al. 2016 ACC/AHA guideline focused update on duration of dual antiplatelet therapy in patients with coronary artery disease: A report of the American College of Cardiology/American Heart Association Task Force on clinical practice guidelines: An update of the 2011 ACCF/AHA/SCAI guideline for percutaneous coronary intervention, 2011 ACCF/AHA guideline

for coronary artery bypass graft surgery, 2012 ACC/AHA/ACP/AATS/PCNA/SCAI/STS guideline for the diagnosis and management of patients with stable ischemic heart disease, 2013 ACCF/AHA guideline for the management of st-elevation myocardial infarction, 2014 AHA/ACC guideline for the management of patients with non-st-elevation acute coronary syndromes, and 2014 ACC/AHA guideline on perioperative cardiovascular evaluation and management of patients undergoing non-cardiac surgery. Circulation 2016;134(10):e123–55.

116.   Zakko L, Rustagi T, Douglas M, et al. No benefit from platelet transfusion for gastrointestinal bleeding in patients taking antiplatelet agents. Clin Gastroenterol Hepatol 2017;15(1):46–52.

117.   Sung JJ, Lau JY, Ching JY, et al. Continuation of low-dose aspirin therapy in peptic ulcer bleeding: A randomized trial. Ann Intern Med 2010;152:1–9.

118.   Malik AH, Yandrapalli S, Shetty SS, et al. Meta-analysis of dual antiplatelet therapy versus monotherapy with P2Y12 inhibitors in patients after percutaneous coronary intervention. Am J Cardiol 2020; 127:25–9.

119.   Kim BK, Hong SJ, Cho YH, et al. Effect of ticagrelor monotherapy vs ticagrelor with aspirin on major bleeding and cardiovascular events in patients with acute coronary syndrome: The TICO randomized clinical trial. JAMA 2020;323(23):2407–16.

120.   Douketis JD, Spyropoulos AC, Kaatz S, et al. Perioperative bridging anticoagulation in patients with atrial fibrillation. N Engl J Med 2015;373:823–33.

121.   Kovacs MJ, Wells PS, Anderson DR, et al. Postoperative low molecular weight heparin bridging treatment for patients at high risk of arterial thromboembolism (PERIOP2): Double blind randomised controlled trial. BMJ 2021;373:n1205.

122.   Sengupta N, Feuerstein JD, Jairath V, Shergill AK, Strate LL, Wong RJ, Wan D. Management of Patients With Acute Lower Gastrointestinal Bleeding: An Updated ACG Guideline. Am J Gastroenterol 2023 Feb 1;118(2):208-231.

123.   Oakland K, Jairath V, Uberoi R, et al. Derivation and validation of a novel risk score for safe discharge after acute lower gastrointestinal bleeding: a modelling study. Lancet Gastroenterol Hepatol. 2017;2(9):635-643.

124.   Oakland K, Kothiwale S, Forehand T, et al. External validation of the Oakland score to assess safe hospital discharge among adult patients with acute lower gastrointestinal bleeding in the US. JAMA Netw Open 2020; 3(7): :e209630.

125.   Chan FK, Leung Ki EL, Wong GL, et al. Risks of bleeding recurrence and cardiovascular events with continued aspirin use after lower gastrointestinal hemorrhage. Gastroenterology 2016;151(2):271–7.

126.   Smith SR, Murray D, Pockney PG, et al. Tranexamic acid for lower GI hemorrhage: A randomized placebo-controlled clinical trial. Dis Colon Rectum 2018;61(1):99–106.

127.   Roberts I, Shakur-Still H, Afolabi A, et al. Effects of a high-dose 24-h infusion of tranexamic acid on death and thromboembolic events in patients with acute gastrointestinal bleeding (HALT-IT): An international randomised, double-blind, placebo-controlled trial. Lancet 2020;395(10241):1927–36.

128.   Jensen DM. Diagnosis and treatment of definitive diverticular hemorrhage (DDH). Am J Gastroenterol 2018;113(11):1570–3.

129.   Umezawa S, Nagata N, Arimoto J, et al. Contrast-enhanced CT for colonic diverticular bleeding before colonoscopy: A prospective multicenter study. Radiology 2018;288(3):755–61.

130.   Koh FH, Soong J, Lieske B, et al. Does the timing of an invasive mesenteric angiography following a positive CT mesenteric angiography make a difference? Int J Colorectal Dis 2015;30(1):57–61.

131.   Jensen DM, Machicado GA, Jutabha R, et al. Urgent colonoscopy for the diagnosis and treatment of severe diverticular hemorrhage. N Engl J Med 2000;342(2):78–82.

132.   Ron-Tal Fisher O, Gralnek IM, Eisen GM, et al. Endoscopic hemostasis is rarely used for hematochezia: A population-based study from the Clinical Outcomes Research Initiative National Endoscopic Database. Gastrointest Endosc 2014;79(2):317–25.

133.   Tsay C, Shung D, Stemmer Frumento K, et al. Early colonoscopy does not improve outcomes of patients with lower gastrointestinal bleeding: Systematic review of randomized trials. Clin Gastroenterol Hepatol 2020; 18(8):1696–703.

134.   Kato M. Endoscopic therapy for acute diverticular bleeding. Clin Endosc. 2019;52(5):419-425.

135.   Nagata N, Niikura R, Ishii N, et al. Cumulative evidence for reducing recurrence of colonic diverticular bleeding using endoscopic clipping versus band ligation: Systematic review and meta-analysis. J Gastroenterol Hepatol 2021;36(7):1738–43.

136.   KobayashiK,NagataN, FurumotoY, et al. Effectiveness and adverse events of endoscopic clipping versus band ligation for colonic diverticular hemorrhage: A large-scale multicenter cohort study. Endoscopy 2022;54(08):735–44.

137.   Brandt L, Feuerstadt P, Longstreth G, Boley SJ. ACG clinical guideline: epidemiology, risk factors, patterns of presentation, diagnosis, and management of colon ischemia (CI). Am J Gastroenterol. 2015;110:18-44.

138.   Brandt LJ, Feuerstadt P, Blaszka MC. Anatomic patterns, patient characteristics, and clinical outcomes in ischemic colitis: a study of 313 cases supported by histology. Am J Gastroenterol 2010;105:2245–2252

139.   Montoro MA, Brandt LJ, Santolaria S et al. Clinical patterns and outcomes of ischaemic colitis: results of the Working Group for the Study of Ischaemic Colitis in Spain (CIE study). Scand J Gastroenterol 2011;46:236–246.

140.   Wolff JH, Rubin A, Potter JD et al. Clinical significance of colonoscopic findings associated with colonic thickening on computed tomography: is colonoscopy warranted when thickening is detected? J Clin Gastroenterol 2008;42:472–475.

6-MP   6-mercaptopurine

ACG   American College of Gastroenterology

ALT   Alanine transaminase

ANCA   Anti-neutrophil cytoplasmic antibodies

AI   Artificial intelligence

ASCA   Anti-saccharomyces cerevisiae antibodies

AST   Aspartate transaminase

ATI   Antibiodies to infliximab

AVM   Arteriovenous malformations

AZA   Azathioprine

BMI   Body mass index

CDAI   Crohn's Disease Activty Index

CDC   Centers for Disease Control and Prevention

CIR   Controlled ileal-release

CMV   Cytomegalovirus

CRP   C-reactive protein

CTA   Computed tomographic angiography

CTE   Computed tomography enterography

ED   Emergency department

ERCP   Endoscopic retrograde cholangiopancreatography

ESR   Erythrocyte sedimentation rate

EUS   Endoscopic ultrasound

Hgb   Hemoglobin

HIV   Human immunodeficiency virus

IBD   Inflammatory bowel disease

IBS   Irritable bowel syndrome

ICU   Intensive care unit

JCV   John Cunningham virus

MRE   Magnetic resonance enterography
MTX   Methotrexate
NG   Nasogastric
NSAID   Non-steroidal anti-inflammatory drug
PML   progressive multifocal leukoencephalopathy
SIBO   small intestinal bacterial overgrowth
TB   tuberculosis
UC   ulcerative colitis
VR   Virtual reality